Models of Care in Women's Health

Edited by
Tahir Mahmood, **Allan Templeton**
and **Charnjit Dhillon**

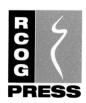

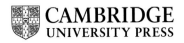

Shaftesbury Road, Cambridge CB2 8EA, United Kingdom

One Liberty Plaza, 20th Floor, New York, NY 10006, USA

477 Williamstown Road, Port Melbourne, VIC 3207, Australia

314–321, 3rd Floor, Plot 3, Splendor Forum, Jasola District Centre, New Delhi – 110025, India

103 Penang Road, #05–06/07, Visioncrest Commercial, Singapore 238467

Cambridge University Press is part of Cambridge University Press & Assessment,
a department of the University of Cambridge.

We share the University's mission to contribute to society through the pursuit of
education, learning and research at the highest international levels of excellence.

www.cambridge.org
Information on this title: www.cambridge.org/9781906985189

First published 2009

A catalogue record for this publication is available from the British Library

ISBN   978-1-906-98518-9   Paperback

A machine-readable catalogue record for this publication can be obtained from the British
Library [www.bl.uk/catalogue/listings.html]

Published by the **RCOG Press** at the
Royal College of Obstetricians and Gynaecologists
27 Sussex Place, Regent's Park
London NW1 4RG

Registered Charity No. 213280

RCOG Press Editor: Jane Moody
Design & typesetting: FiSH Books, Enfield

Contents

About the authors

Alison Bigrigg FRCOG
Director
The Sandyford Initiative, Glasgow, Scotland, UK

Audrey Brown MRCOG
Consultant in Sexual and Reproductive Healthcare
The Sandyford Initiative, Glasgow, Scotland, UK

Margaret E Cruickshank FRCOG
Consultant Gynaecologist
Aberdeen Royal Infirmary, Scotland, UK

Alfred Cutner FRCOG
Consultant Gynaecologist
Elizabeth Garrett Anderson and Obstetric Hospital, University College London Hospital, UK

Feroza Dawood MRCOG
Consultant Obstetrician and Gynaecologist
Liverpool Women's Hospital, Liverpool, UK

Charnjit Dhillon
Director of Standards
Royal College of Obstetricians and Gynaecologists, London, UK

Edmond Edi-Osagie MRCOG
Consultant in Obstetrics and Gynaecologist
St. Mary's Hospital, Manchester, UK

Leroy Edozien FRCOG
Consultant Obstetrician and Gynaecologist
St. Mary's Hospital, Manchester, UK

Roy Farquharson FRCOG
Consultant Gynaecologist
Liverpool Women's Hospital, Liverpool, UK

Robert Freeman FRCOG
Consultant Obstetrician and Gynaecologist
Derriford Hospital, Plymouth, UK

Ailsa Gebbie FRCOG
Consultant in Community Gynaecology
NHS Lothian Family Planning Services, Edinburgh, UK

Mark Hamilton FRCOG
Consultant Gynaecologist
Aberdeen Maternity Hospital, Scotland, UK

Salma Kayani MRCOG
Clinical Fellow in Advanced Minimal Access Surgery
Elizabeth Garrett Anderson and Obstetric Hospital, University College
London Hospital, UK

Henry Kitchener FRCOG
Professor of Gynaecological Oncology
School of Cancer and Imaging Sciences, University of Manchester, UK

Mary Ann Lumsden FRCOG
Professor of Medical Education and Gynaecology
University of Glasgow, Glasgow, UK

Kay McAllister MRCOG
Consultant in Sexual and Reproductive Health
The Sandyford Initiative, Glasgow, Scotland, UK

Gavin MacNab FRCOG
Lead Consultant and Clinical Director in Obstetrics and Gynaecology
Sunderland Royal Hospital, Tyne and Wear, UK

Tahir Mahmood FRCOG
Consultant Obstetrician and Gynaecologist, Vice-President of Standards
Forth Park Maternity Hospital, Scotland, Royal College of Obstetricians
and Gynaecologists, London, UK

Arti Matah
Specialist Registrar
St George's Hospital and Medical School, London, UK

Ash Monga MRCOG
Consultant Urogynaecologist
Princess Anne Hospital, Southampton, UK

Andy Nordin
Consultant Gynaecological Oncologist and Clinical Adviser for Gynaecology, NHS Improvement–Cancer
East Kent Gynaecological Oncology Centre UK

Kamal Ojha MRCOG
Consultant in Obstetrics and Gynaecology
St George's Hospital and Medical School, London, UK

Georgios Pandis MRCOG
Consultant Obstetrician and Gynaecologist
Elizabeth Garrett Anderson and Obstetric Hospital, University Hospital, UK

Charles Redman FRCOG
Consultant Gynaecological Oncologist
University Hospital of North Staffordshire

Margaret Rees
Reader in Reproductive Medicine
John Radcliffe Hospital, Oxford, UK

Mahmood Shafi FRCOG
Consultant Gynaecological Surgeon and Oncologist
Addenbrooke's Hospital, Cambridge, UK

Allan Templeton FRCOG
Clinical Director, Office for Research and Clinical Audit
Royal College of Obstetricians and Gynaecology, London, UK

John Tidy FRCOG
Consultant Gynaecological Oncologist
Royal Hallamshire Hospital, Sheffield, UK

Richard Todd MRCOG
Consultant Gynaecological Oncologist
University Hospital North Staffordshire, Stoke-on-Trent, UK

Lilantha Wedisinghe
Specialist Trainee in Obstetrics and Gynaecology
Glasgow Royal Infirmary, Glasgow, UK

Abbreviations

AEPU	Association of Early Pregnancy Units
AIDS	autoimmune deficiency syndrome
ATSM	Advanced Training Skills Module
BASHH	British Association for Sexual Health and HIV
BFS	British Fertility Society
BGCS	British Gynaecological Cancer Society
BSCCP	British Society for Colposcopy and Cervical Pathology
BSGE	British Society for Gynaecological Endoscopy
BSUG	British Society of Urogynaecology
CIN	cervical intraepithelial neoplasia
CLRN	comprehensive research network
CNST	Clinical Negligence Scheme for Trusts
CQUIN	commissioning for quality and innovation
DFSRH	Diploma of the FSRH
DNA	deoxyribonucleic acid
EGGS	expectations, goal setting, goal achievement and satisfaction
FIGO	International Federation of Gynecology and Obstetrics
FRSH	Faculty of Sexual and Reproductive Healthcare of the RCOG
GnRHa	gonadotrophin-releasing hormone analogue
GP	general practitioner
hCG	human chorionic gonadotrophin
HFEA	Human Fertilisation and Embryology Authority
HIV	human immunodeficiency syndrome
HPV	human papillomavirus
HRT	hormone replacement therapy
IVF	in vitro fertilisation
LARC	long-acting reversible contraception
LNG-IUS	levonorgestrel-releasing intrauterine system

MEWS	modified early warning scores
MHRA	Medicines and Healthcare products Regulatory Authority
NCIN	National Cancer Intelligence Network
NCRI	National Cancer Research Institute
NHS	National Health Service
NHSCSP	National Health Service Cancer Screening Programme
NHSLA	National Health Service Litigation Authority
NICE	National Institute for Health and Clinical Excellence
NSAIDs	nonsteroidal anti-inflammatory drugs
OHSS	ovarian hyperstimulation syndrome
OSCE	objective structured clinical examination
PMETB	Postgraduate Medical Education and Training Board
PUL	pregnancy of unknown location
QIS	Quality Improvement Scotland
Rh	rhesus
RCOG	Royal College of Obstetricians and Gynaecologists
SIGN	Scottish Intercollegiate Guidelines Network
SHA	strategic health authority
TVU	transvaginal ultrasound
VTE	venous thromboembolism

Preface

Allan Templeton

This book is all about improving the quality of care in gynaecological practice, particularly women's health, recognising that quality in health care is a continuously evolving process. The models of care are rooted in the *Standards for Gynaecology* that have evolved over recent years, derived from clinical guidelines, consensus recommendations and increasingly women's needs. The individual chapters reflect the fact that the main drivers for improvement are clinical effectiveness, and increasing patient expectations. In each area of practice described here, there is recognition that the appropriate clinical response to these drivers is service organisation. Clinicians need to take responsibility not only for managing individual patient conditions but also for developing services which meet patients' needs.

Importantly, this book also reflects the understanding that clinical developments will only come about if clinicians take the initiative to ensure that improvements happen and, at the same time, act in the interests of the total patient population they serve, including, perhaps most importantly, those who have most difficulty accessing services. Clinical governance is the primary responsibility of all consultants in obstetrics and gynaecology and, crucially, this includes the development of effective and responsive clinical services.

It is now accepted that consultants need awareness and knowledge of these issues. The RCOG specialist training curriculum now recognises and emphasises topics such as clinical leadership, service organisation and, perhaps most importantly, multiprofessional working (working in teams). Training which reflects these issues will best meet the future healthcare needs of women.

Service development and, where necessary, reorganisation is thus primarily the responsibility of the relevant lead clinician. Clearly organisational issues will require the support of managers, particularly if there are resource and personnel issues. This, in turn, requires that clinicians will learn to work more effectively with managers, one of the aspirations of the current health service. However, it is striking, in the various developments described in this book, how much can be achieved within current resources and without the need for major additional expense. There will be different approaches, as demonstrated by the different styles used in this book, but the key issue is the patient pathway, with the underlying philosophy of continuous improvement in quality. Patient participation and patient feedback in the development of services should now be taken for granted.

Clinical leadership is the key to success and there is increasing evidence that obstetricians and gynaecologists are more than equal to the tasks in hand and recognise the satisfaction that derives from being associated with clinical development and improvements in the quality of care for women.

CHAPTER 1
Setting the scene

Tahir Mahmood and Charnjit Dhillon

In recent years, there has been an unprecedented emphasis on the quality of clinical care. This has involved three main stakeholders, namely consumers, healthcare providers and commissioners, but increasingly the media has become a vocal partner as well. The perceptions of quality, however, vary among the different stakeholders. Consumers of health care expect an equitable, safe and effective service, available within easy reach. Patients' perception of quality depends largely on personal experience and the overall outcome of their contact with the clinical service. The media has also developed an important role as the patient's champion, by publicising adverse outcomes and poor patient experience, although the fact that the vast majority of patients have a satisfactory or positive outcome is not often emphasised. The Patient's Charter was published to set standards for overall patient care, in particular to provide clear rules for voicing concerns about clinical care, recommending that each unit should have a complaints procedure policy in place for dealing with patients' concerns.[1] The Department of Health's document, *A First Class Service*, outlined a policy of ensuring 'quality' in the National Health Service, suggesting that standards would be set by the National Institute for Health and Clinical Excellence (NICE) and the National Service Framework, delivered via clinical governance, lifelong learning and professional regulation and monitored through the National Performance Framework and national surveys on patients and user experience.[2]

Healthcare providers (doctors, midwives and nurses among others) broadly assess quality of care by measuring outcome indicators, using locally collected information. Most of the established audit systems do not measure patient experience in totality along a care pathway. Several publications have reported that surgical procedures are now becoming safer, with low complication rates. Understandably, it is now largely accepted that clinical episodes will have a satisfactory outcome. The focus has now moved to other markers of quality, such as issues around communication, the local environment (including cleanliness) and a higher degree of specialist input. These quality measures rank high in patient feedback, even higher than satisfaction related to clinical outcomes.

The views of management focus largely on measuring quality of care in terms of financial cost to the trust. They pursue risk-averse strategies to contain costs, although there may also be a need to expand resources on employing clinical risk teams and their training.

The challenge for medical staff is to ensure that risk management strategies, such as the implementation of antibiotic prophylaxis, do result in reducing complications secondary to poor clinical practice. This approach may ultimately save a trust millions of pounds. Similarly, managing the majority of tubal ectopic pregnancies by laparoscopic surgery would not only reduce inpatient days, and thus associated costs, but could also release pressures elsewhere, such as the shortage of inpatient beds.

The philosophy of clinical governance has now been increasingly adopted by NHS organisations to ensure that they continuously strive towards improving the quality of their service and safeguard high standards of care by creating an environment in which excellence in clinical care will flourish. The key objective of the Royal College of Obstetricians and Gynaecologists (RCOG) is to set standards to improve women's health. The College produces guidelines and standards in various formats and these are complemented by the work of other national bodies, such as NICE and the Scottish Intercollegiate Guidelines Network (SIGN). The current portfolio of the RCOG includes over 50 clinical guidelines, opinion papers and good practice series (available on the College's website: www.rcog.org.uk.

The purpose of setting standards is to address variations in care, to prevent inappropriate care and to address issues of inequity which have been reported in the past. Examples include a study in the 1980s of 30 hospitals in the USA which demonstrated up to an eight-fold variation in surgical practice[3] and another study reporting higher rates for hysterectomy in the USA as compared with those in England and Norway.[4] A recent analysis of Hospital Episode Statistics data in England has demonstrated a four-fold regional variation in the rate of endometrial ablations for the management of women presenting with heavy menstrual bleeding.[5] A national survey carried out by the Scottish Programme of Clinical Effectiveness in Reproductive Health on the management of early pregnancy loss showed a wide variation in the care of patients who were offered different types of treatment in 15 Scottish units.[6] All these examples demonstrate the huge challenge ahead.

In 2002, the College published its document, *Clinical Standards: Advice on Planning the Service in Obstetrics and Gynaecology*, which describes 12 standards for core areas of service.[7] This was the first attempt by any Royal College to demonstrate the potential use of guidelines to derive standards. This document has now been superseded by two working party reports, including *Standards for Gynaecology*,[8] which covers 20 key areas of gynaecological care. This document clearly lays out standards for aspects of care in each clinical service. Implementation of care pathways will ultimately help to improve efficiency, reduce costs and improve quality and outcome of care through increased standardisation of practice and better communication between staff, managers and patients.

It is reassuring that quality initiatives are at the top of the National Health Service's agenda. The RCOG is responding to this challenge by taking a lead in developing evidence-based service standards to support local implementation protocols in all areas of gynaecological practice. Implementation of these standards should be supported by undertaking a constantly evolving audit cycle and by having multidisciplinary involvement to measure performance. We need to measure whether standards have been achieved and to identify areas for improvement, if necessary by seeking additional resources, with the ultimate aim of improving standards of care for women, wherever we work. The direction of travel of the NHS is now for a patient-focused and quality-assured service, where patients' experience will influence service delivery models.

There is now a greater emphasis on patient involvement to meet patient needs and expectations. Lord Darzi and his team have set out an ambitious vision in *High Quality Care for All* to improve the quality of care.[9] This vision will be achieved by the development of national quality metrics that will form the basis of commissioning for quality and innovation (CQUIN). At regional level, strategic health authorities (SHAs) will measure a small set of metrics to benchmark organisations and to derive quality indicators. We envisage that the standards developed by the RCOG will underpin the metrics to be developed for the second phase. These initiatives are pivotal in creating a stimulus for developing local care pathways based on standards described in this document and to constantly strive towards enhancement of care. We understand that professional bodies and NICE will be working together in developing a framework for service accreditation using some of the evidence used in our standards document.

The way forward

To implement this ambitious agenda, good communication between clinical staff and management is of paramount importance. The chapters included in this book clearly describe outcome indicators. This College is supportive of informed choice but we also advocate that informed choice should be supported by full and frank discussion between professionals and patients about the potential risks and benefits, as well as the consequences of patient choice. For example, for the management of early pregnancy loss, rather than measuring the percentage of women managed by conservative, medical or surgical options, a more relevant approach would be to measure how many women received their preferred management and whether they had adequate explanation.

Lord Darzi's report recognises that there remains unacceptable variation in the quality of care across the country.[9] A central purpose of this book is to define a road map of quality service anchored in clinical effectiveness, patient safety and the patient's experience. Darzi also singles out professionalism as a vital lever for raising standards.[10] It is now up to us professionals to take this exceptional opportunity and make it work for patients. This volume seeks to offer pragmatic advice for the introduction of evidence-based clinical pathways, complemented by outcome measurements to safeguard patient safety. Standards of care will only improve if all outcome measures are regularly collected and demonstrate evidence of enhanced care with a strategy of continuous improvement in place. By setting up such a monitoring system, each service unit can assess its progress against national benchmarks. The information technology revolution is making it possible to capture a previously unimaginable range of information about the inputs, processes and outcomes of health care.

We are very grateful to the many contributors and experts for their thoughtful presentations. We hope trainees, clinicians, managers and commissioners of services will find this text of practical value. Our responsibility as clinicians is not to just see patients but also to support doctors in training and to provide, organise and review clinical services, so that they remain equitable and safe but with best possible outcomes for women seeking gynaecological care.

References

1. Great Britain, Scottish Office. *The Patient's Charter: A Charter for Health.* Edinburgh: Scottish office; 1991.
2. Department of Health. *A First Class Service: Quality in the New NHS.* London: The Stationery Office; 1998.
3. Coulter A, McPherson K, Vessey M. Do British Women undergo too many or too few hysterectomies? *Soc Sci Med* 1988;27:987–94.
4   McPherson K, Wennberg JE, Hovind OB, Clifford P. Small areas variations in the use of common surgical procedures: an international comparison of New England, England and Norway. *N Engl J Med* 1982;307:1310–14.
5. Cromwell D, Mahmood TA, Templeton A, Vander Meulen JH. Surgery for menorrhagia within English regions: variations in rates of endometrial ablation and hysterectomy. *BJOG* 2009;116:1373–9.
6. Scottish Programme for Clinical Effectiveness in Reproductive Health (SPCERH) [www.nhshealthquality.org/nhsqis/3803.html].
7. Royal College of Obstetricians and Gynaecologists. *Clinical Standards: Advice on Planning the Service in Obstetrics and Gynaecology.* London: RCOG Press; 2002.
8. Royal College of Obstetricians and Gynaecologists. *Standards for Gynaecology.* London: RCOG Press; 2008 [www.rcog.org.uk/womens-health/clinical-guidance/standards-gynaecology].
9. Department of Health. *A High Quality Care for All: NHS Next Stage Review.* CM7432. London: The Stationery Office; 2008
10. Royal College of Physicians. *Doctors in Society. Medical Professionalism in a Changing World.* London: RCP; 2008.

CHAPTER 2

Early pregnancy loss, including ectopic pregnancy and recurrent miscarriage

Roy Farquharson and Feroza Dawood

Key points

✓ All women with early pregnancy complications should be evaluated in a dedicated early pregnancy unit.
✓ Management should be conducted by trained and competent staff.
✓ Adequate facilities should exist to perform scans and for the measurement of serum beta human chorionic gonadotrophin levels.
✓ Algorithms should be in place to guide the management of spontaneous and recurrent miscarriage and ectopic pregnancy.
✓ Women should be offered an informed choice of management options.
✓ Women should be furnished with written information in non-medical language.
✓ A quiet room conducive to breaking bad news should be located away from the work area.
✓ Bereavement counselling should be offered to all women who suffer a pregnancy loss.
✓ Adherence to local and national standards should be audited regularly.

Introduction

Early pregnancy problems form a major part of all gynaecological emergencies. Early pregnancy loss before 12 weeks of gestation is a common event, which causes a great deal of distress to women and their partners alike. Approximately one in five pregnancies will end in pregnancy loss, which represents a considerable burden on individuals and their healthcare providers.

In the past, women were admitted to the emergency receiving ward and waited for a considerable length of time before undergoing ultrasound scan and clinical assessment. With the appearance of early pregnancy assessment units, an increasing number of women are being assessed and managed as outpatient attenders. The advent of high-resolution transvaginal ultrasound, coupled with the improved access to serum human chorionic gonadotrophin (hCG) measurements, has allowed the development of models of care and improved delivery of care.

Within the UK, the number of early pregnancy assessment units has increased to the extent that over 200 active units are registered with the Association of Early Pregnancy Units (AEPU). The AEPU has set out, since its inception in 2001, to improve the standards of early pregnancy care and to provide a clearer pathway for the patient's journey.[1]

In recent years, ultrasound diagnosis and improved understanding of problems related to early pregnancy have led to the introduction of medical and expectant management of miscarriage and selected cases of ectopic pregnancy.

The service user's view

The model of care for all early pregnancy events and complications is best composed around the woman's journey. This provides the timeline base along which the core standards of care elements, care pathways and clinical protocols (Figure 2.1) can support the care provision for 'best patient experience'.

Feedback from support organisations such as the Miscarriage Association, the Ectopic Pregnancy Trust and the AEPU suggests that women want prompt and sensitive treatment of early pregnancy problems and a full explanation of management choices, which should be supplemented with easy-to-read patient information leaflets.

Clinical standards and national guidelines

All women with early pregnancy problems should have prompt access to a dedicated early pregnancy unit that provides efficient, evidence-based care with access to appropriate information and counselling. The

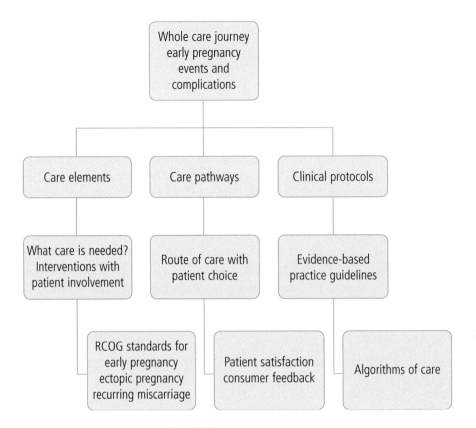

Figure 2.1 Overview of clinical model for early pregnancy

National Service Framework recommends that all women should have access to an early pregnancy unit that should be easily available. Ideally, these services should also be directly accessible to general practitioners. An ideal aspiration would be a choose-and-book system that is easily available to women. At all times, women should be supported in making informed choices about their care and management. These choices should be supplemented by easy-to-read information leaflets. Appropriate follow-up systems should be in place to facilitate repeat scans or blood tests.

The core and aspirational standards for each clinical event within early pregnancy should drive the care provision and should identify strongly with established peer-reviewed standards published by the RCOG.[2]

Service model for the management of miscarriage

Diagnosis

The diagnosis of miscarriage is based on a well-recognised peer-reviewed protocol as summarised in Figure 2.2.[3] Ultrasound diagnosis is used universally in the presence of an intrauterine sac and is confirmed by serial observation wherever doubt exists as to the viability of the pregnancy (pregnancy of uncertain viability). The initial diagnosis of fetal loss (loss of previously documented fetal heart activity) should always be confirmed by a second independent trained observer. Many women in this situation request a subsequent scan to confirm the original finding and their request should be supported.

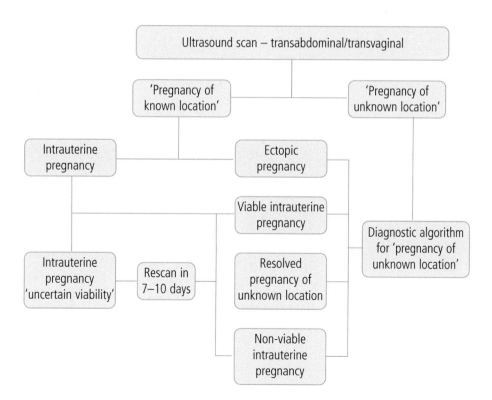

Figure 2.2 Basic diagnostic algorithm for early pregnancy loss

Management

In recent years, ultrasound diagnosis and improved understanding of problems related to early pregnancy has led to the introduction of medical and expectant management of miscarriage and selected cases of ectopic pregnancy in addition to the traditional surgical option (Figure 2.3). Randomised controlled trials have provided evidence-based practice.

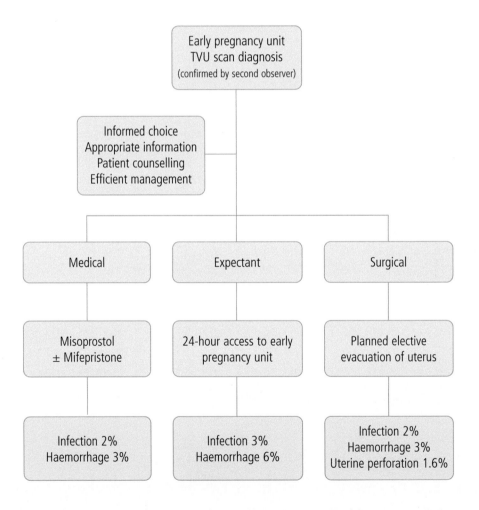

Figure 2.3 Management of miscarriage (source: RCOG Green-top Guideline No. 25, 2006)

Patient choice has emerged as a powerful selector for the treatment of miscarriage. The mission statement from the AEPU has the patient at the centre of all activity and the multidisciplinary care structure reflects the multi-tasking approach of care providers: 'All women with early pregnancy problems will have prompt access to a dedicated early pregnancy unit that provides efficient evidence-based care with access to appropriate information and counselling. At all times women will be supported in making informed choices about their care and management'.

Medical management

The drugs used for medical management of a miscarriage include an antiprogesterone, oral mifepristone (200 mg) with a prostaglandin such as misoprostol administered vaginally (200 micrograms × 2 or 400 micrograms × 2).

The original prostaglandin E_1 analogue used for abortion procedures is gemeprost. It is effective in 95% of cases in combination with mifepristone at less than 63 days of amenorrhoea. The alternative E_1 analogue, misoprostol, may be given orally or vaginally and it is most effective if administered vaginally (95% compared with 87%, respectively).[1] The main advantages over gemeprost are that it does not require refrigeration, it is cheaper and can be administered orally or vaginally.

Contraindications to medical management are shown in Table 2.1.

Table 2.1 Contraindications to medical management of early pregnancy loss

Absolute	Adrenal insufficiency
	Long-term glucocorticoid therapy
	Haemoglobinopathies or anticoagulant therapy
	Anaemia (haemoglobin < 10 g/dl)
	Porphyria
	Mitral stenosis
	Glaucoma
	Nonsteroidal anti-inflammatory drug ingestion in previous 48 hours
Relative	Hypertension
	Severe asthma

Varying rates of efficacy have been quoted with medical management in non-viable pregnancies. The efficacy is greatest for those pregnancies of less than 10 weeks or with a sac diameter of less than 24 mm (92–94%).

Figure 2.4 shows the protocol for the medical management of miscarriage.[3]

Surgical evacuation of uterus for miscarriage

Surgical evacuation is preferably managed on a daycase basis unless there is heavy bleeding, when the woman should be admitted urgently to the gynaecology ward.

Have a local unit protocol for admission system with a patient pathway clearly described.

Give the patient information on the admission procedure, including appropriate patient information leaflet(s).

Explain the surgical procedure and obtain written consent with a doctor familiar with the procedure. Mention rare anaesthetic and uncommon surgical risks involved, such as uterine perforation (1%), cervical tears, intra-abdominal trauma (0.1%), intrauterine adhesions, haemorrhage and infection.

Arrange for measurement of haemoglobin concentration and determination of ABO and Rh blood groups. Anti-D immunoglobulin should be given to all non-sensitised Rh-negative women undergoing surgical evacuation.

All at-risk women (usually women under the age of 25 years) undergoing surgical evacuation for miscarriage should be screened for *Chlamydia trachomatis*.[4] Alternatively, prescribe prophylactic doxycycline 100 mg orally twice daily for 7 days and metronidazole 1 g rectally at the time of surgical evacuation according to the local protocol.

Ensure that products of conception are seen at evacuation.

Current recommendations are that all tissue obtained at a surgical evacuation for miscarriage should be sent for histology examination. The reasons are:

- to diagnose molar pregnancy
- to exclude ectopic pregnancy if chorionic tissue is found on histology.

A follow-up appointment is usually not required after a surgical evacuation.

- Ensure that the patient has read information leaflet.
- Ask if she has any questions.
- Follow local early pregnancy unit protocol.
- Obtain written consent for mifepristone and misoprostol administration.
- Arrange blood tests:
  - measurement of haemoglobin concentration
  - determination of ABO and rhesus (Rh) blood groups with screening for red-cell antibodies.
- Anti-D immunoglobulin should be given to all non-sensitised Rh-negative women undergoing medical evacuation.
- In the case of a pregnancy occurring with an intrauterine contraceptive device in place, the device should be removed before administration of mifepristone.
- Prescribe **mifepristone 200 mg orally**.
- Arrange attendance 48 (36–72) hours after mifepristone administration.
- Inform the woman regarding the length of stay. Observe for 3–6 hours after administration of prostaglandin and discharge if she is clinically well.
- Women with gestations of:
  - less than 9 weeks on scan have only one insertion of misoprostol 800 micrograms vaginally. Misoprostol tablets are administered vaginally by the woman or clinician. If miscarriage has not occurred 4 hours after administration of misoprostol, a further dose of misoprostol 400 micrograms may be administered orally or vaginally.
  - 9 weeks or above on scan can have a maximum of four further doses of misoprostol 400 micrograms at 3-hourly intervals, vaginally or orally depending on the amount of bleeding and woman's preference.
- Prescribe prostaglandins (misoprostol 800-microgram tablets/gemeprost1mg) vaginally and metronidazole 1 g rectally.
- Prescribe doxycycline 100 mg twice daily for 7 days with co-dydramol 2 tablets four times a day for 1 week for the woman to take home after the procedure.
- Inform her that, if she bleeds heavily, an evacuation may be required and she should be prepared to stay overnight if necessary.
- Women may or may not pass products of conception while on the ward. They should be advised of what to expect when they go home and not referred to the early pregnancy unit for a scan before their follow-up appointment, as most of them will miscarry at a later stage after discharge from the hospital.
- Any products that are obtained should be sent for histological examination to exclude a molar pregnancy or arrange a urine pregnancy test 3–4 weeks later.
- Give patient information on:
  - admission to the gynaecology ward
  - medical management of non-viable pregnancy:
    - ⇨ what to expect and the likely amount of blood loss
    - ⇨ what analgesics to take
    - ⇨ what sort of sanitary protection to use.
- Arrange follow-up in the early pregnancy unit **3 weeks** later (to avoid further appointments if products of conception are seen at an early scan or in a surgical intervention).
- Give contact telephone numbers for early pregnancy unit, gynaecology emergency room, ward.

Figure 2.4 Protocol for medical management of miscarriage[4]

Give information on 'What you may need to know after a miscarriage'. There should be information on counselling if required in the future.

Expectant management of miscarriage

A significant number of women prefer expectant management and it may be continued as long as the woman is willing, provided that there are no signs of infection such as:

- vaginal discharge
- excessive bleeding
- pyrexia
- abdominal pain.

Conservative management requires:

- motivation and preparation
- a thorough explanation of:
  - what to expect: the likely amount of blood loss and pain
  - what analgesics to be taken
  - what sort of sanitary protection to be used
- satisfactory answers to any questions and doubts
- reassurance that the risk of infection is negligible (less than 3%)
- a contact number, which should be available 24 hours to ring if there are any problems such as very heavy loss or severe pain (an adequately informed and reassured patient is less likely to contact for any further advice)
- a follow-up appointment for confirmation that the miscarriage is complete and to assess whether she has any pain or bleeding
- an information leaflet to support the verbal explanation, such as that provided by the RCOG.[5]

Success rates are higher with prolonged follow-up. Follow-up scans may be arranged at 2-weekly intervals, until a diagnosis of complete miscarriage is made. However if the woman requests a surgical or medical method at any stage, her request should be accommodated. In general, 90% of women miscarry within 3 weeks. Only a small percentage of women may go up to 6–8 weeks.

In the absence of clinically different relevant differences in safety, noninvasive treatment modalities can now be offered with confidence to women with first-trimester miscarriage who wish to avoid surgical evacuation. This is important, since freedom of treatment choice improves quality of life for these women. Infection rates (2–3%) after expectant, medical and surgical management are not significantly different and are reassuringly low.[6,7]

Ectopic pregnancy

As ectopic pregnancy is a life-threatening condition, women should have prompt access to a dedicated early pregnancy unit providing efficient management and patient counselling. Units should have a protocol in place for conducting a pregnancy test and performing transvaginal ultrasound in women of reproductive age with amenorrhea associated with abdominal pain. Access to serial serum hCG laboratory measurements is mandatory for efficient diagnosis, surveillance and monitoring. All units should have clear guidelines in place for the management of pregnancies of unknown location. All early pregnancy assessment units should have in place clear guidelines for the management of pregnancies of unknown location, based on the RCOG Green-top Guideline No. 21: *The Management of Tubal Pregnancy.*[8] A clear explanation of surgical, medical and expectant management options should be given, depending on the clinical scenario and local availability.

Service model for ectopic pregnancy

Medical management

Many agents, including prostaglandins, mifepristone, potassium chloride and dactinomycin, have all been used for the medical management of ectopic pregnancy. The most commonly used drug is, however, methotrexate. A single injection of methotrexate is well tolerated and is effective. Published studies have shown a success rate varying from 52–94% for single-dose methotrexate.

Methotrexate is a folic acid-antagonist (anti-metabolite) which prevents the growth of rapidly dividing cells by interfering with DNA synthesis. It can be administered systematically (intravenously, intramuscularly or orally). It is most commonly given according to a single-dose protocol, which involves a single intramuscular dose of 50 mg/m^2.

Inclusion criteria

- Haemodynamically stable.
- Indications:
    - unruptured tubal or other ectopic pregnancy (diagnosed with serial hCG and transvaginal ultrasound)
    - persistent trophoblast after salpingotomy
- An ectopic pregnancy with serum hCG less than 3000 iu.
- An ectopic pregnancy with serum hCG value less than 1000 iu/litre should have repeat serum hCG within 48 hours if the patient remains haemodynamically stable:
    - the treatment should begin if levels are plateauing
    - if levels are rising, you must exclude intrauterine pregnancy before starting treatment.
- Normal liver function, urea and electrolytes and full blood count.

Exclusion criteria

- Any evidence of intraperitoneal haemorrhage: that is, haemoperitoneum on transvaginal ultrasound scan.
- Any hepatic dysfunction, thrombocytopenia (platelet count less than 100,000), blood dyscrasia (white cell count less than 2000 cells/cm^3).
- Difficulty or unwillingness of patient for prolonged follow-up (average follow-up 35 days).
- Ectopic mass greater than 3.5 mm
- The presence of cardiac activity in an ectopic pregnancy.
- Women taking concurrent corticosteroid therapy.

A treatment protocol for ectopic pregnancy is shown in Figure 2.5.

- Discuss options for management: expectant, surgical or medical.
- Satisfy eligibility and exclusion criteria.
- Counsel the woman and explain treatment protocol. Give information leaflet.
- Take height and weight.
- Prescribe methotrexate (Table 2.2).
- Organise baseline blood tests: full blood count, blood group, liver function and urea and electrolytes.
- Send prescription with the height and weight documented to pharmacy to make up the drug.
- Check blood results, prescribe anti-D immunoglobulin if Rh-negative.
- Give methotrexate intramuscularly in buttock or lateral thigh. The empty syringe or needle should be placed in a separate sharp safe that is labelled 'Cytotoxic waste for special incineration'.
- The patient should rest for up to 1 hour. Check for any local reaction. If a local reaction is noted, consider giving an antihistamine or steroid cream (very rare).
- Arrange follow-up in early pregnancy unit.

Figure 2.5 Treatment protocol for ectopic pregnancy

Information for clinicians

- Up to 75% of women may complain of pain on days 3–7 (thought to be due to tubal miscarriage).
- hCG levels may initially rise days 1–4 (up to 86% of women).
- Mean time to resolution is 35 days.
- A second dose of methotrexate may be given at 7 days if hCG levels fail to fall by more than 15% between day 4 and day 7 (3–27% in published literature); 14% of medically treated women will require more than one dose of methotrexate).

Table 2.2 Methotrexate single-dose regimen

Day	Management
0	Serum hCG, full blood count, urea and electrolytes, liver function tests, group and save
1	Serum hCG Intramuscular methotrexate 50 mg/m^2
4	Serum hCG
7	Serum hCG, full blood count, liver function tests Second dose of methotrexate if hCG decrease less than 15% days 4–7 If hCG decrease greater than 15% repeat hCG weekly until less than 12 units/litre

- Risk of tubal rupture is 7% and the risk remains while there is persistent hCG. Folinic acid rescue is not required for the single-dose regimen.
- Avoid vaginal examination. Transvaginal ultrasound scan may be undertaken during first treatment week or subsequently if clinically indicated.
- Transvaginal ultrasound should be used to monitor completeness of resolution of an ectopic pregnancy after hCG values are normalised.
- Ovarian cysts may be found in the post-treatment phase, which undergo spontaneous resolution.

Information for patients

- Medical treatment for ectopic pregnancy is now well established and approximately 90% of women do not require further surgery. Methotrexate is used for a variety of clinical conditions, such as psoriasis, as well as for malignancies.
- Prolonged follow-up is required with blood tests until serum hCG level is below 20 iu/litre.
- A further dose of methotrexate may be necessary.
- 75% of women experience abdominal pain following treatment, which is due to the drug acting on tubal pregnancy. It usually occurs on days 3–7.
- Pregnancy should be avoided for 3 months after methotrexate has been given, because of a possible teratogenic effect – advice should be to use a reliable barrier or hormonal contraception.
- Side effects of the drug are minimal but may include nausea, vomiting and stomatitis.
- Maintain ample fluid intake.
- Avoid alcohol or folic acid-containing vitamins during treatment.
- Avoid sexual intercourse until resolution of the ectopic pregnancy.
- Avoid exposure to sunlight.

Outcome

- 90% successful treatment with single-dose regimen.
- Recurrent ectopic pregnancy rate 10–20%.
- Tubal patency approximately 80%.

Surgical management of ectopic pregnancy

Laparoscopy or laparotomy?
Advantages and disadvantages of laparoscopy for managing ectopic pregnancy are shown in Table 2.3. A laparoscopic approach is superior to a laparotomy in terms of recovery from surgery.

Laparotomy is to be preferred:

- in cases with haemorrhagic shock
- where a surgeon has inadequate experience of operative laparoscopy
- where there is a lack of equipment and instruments.

Do what is safe in the circumstances

Salpingectomy or salpingostomy?
In a meta-analysis of nine good-quality comparative studies:

- there was no significant difference in the subsequent intrauterine pregnancy between salpingotomy and salpingectomy groups (53% compared with 49.3%)
- the recurrent ectopic pregnancy rate was higher after salpingotomy (15%) than after salpingectomy (10%)
- persistence of trophoblast was noted in 4.8–11.0% of salpingotomy cases; hence the need to monitor hCG postoperatively
- in contrast, almost no cases of persistence of trophoblast followed salpingectomy; there is no need to measure hCG in the postoperative period following salpingectomy.

Table 2.3 Advantages and disadvantages of laparoscopy for ectopic pregnancy

Advantages	Shorter hospital stay (1–2 days)
	Significantly less blood loss
	Less adhesion formation
	Lower analgesia requirements
	Quicker postoperative recovery time
	Recurrent ectopic pregnancy rate lower (5%) than after laparotomy (16.6%)
	Subsequent intrauterine pregnancy rate better (70%) than after laparotomy
Disadvantages	Increased risk of bowel or vascular damage

In the presence of a healthy contralateral tube, there is no clear evidence that salpingotomy should be used in preference to salpingectomy. Laparoscopic salpingotomy should be considered as the primary treatment when managing tubal pregnancy in the presence of contralateral tubal disease and the desire for future fertility.[8]

Discuss with the patient treatment and options of conserving or removing the tube

Follow-up regimen after salpingotomy

While the trophoblast remains in the tube it has a capacity to rupture. Follow up at weekly intervals until serum hCG level is less than 5 iu. If hCG level is rising or plateauing, consider further treatment with methotrexate or surgery if hCG levels greater than 5000 iu. Suturing the salpingotomy lesion provides no benefit.

Outcome after conservative surgery in women with one tube

- Recurrent ectopic pregnancy rate 20.5%
- Intrauterine pregnancy rate 54%

Conservative surgery may be appropriate but only if the woman is aware of the risk involved. Salpingectomy followed by in vitro fertilisation is an alternative therapy in such cases. An algorithm for the management of suspected ectopic pregnancy is shown in Figure 2.6.

Recurrent miscarriage

Recurrent miscarriage affects about 1% of couples. Maternal age and the number of previous losses are two important factors in determining future prognosis. Although the pathophysiology remains unknown in almost 50% of cases, structural uterine abnormalities, chromosomal anomalies and maternal thrombophilia has been directly associated with recurrent miscarriage.[9]

All early pregnancy units or recurrent miscarriage clinics should have a clearly defined protocol for the investigation of women with recurrent miscarriage.[10]

Recurring miscarriage is defined as three consecutive early pregnancy losses (empty-sac type) or two consecutive fetal losses (loss of fetal heart activity following ultrasound confirmation). The appearance of either of

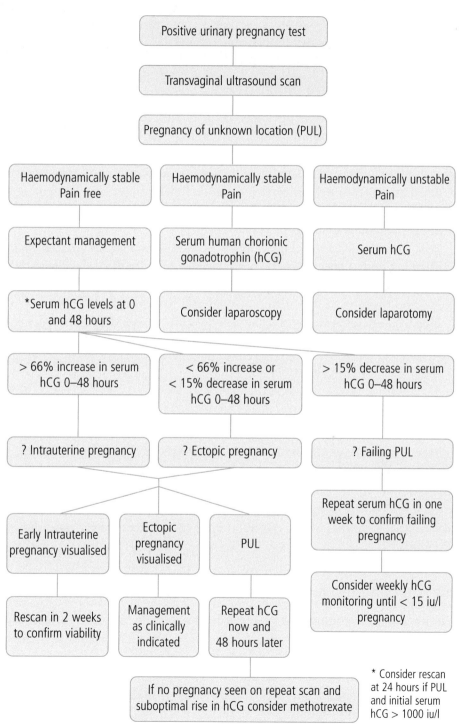

Figure 2.6 Suggested algorithm for management of suspected ectopic pregnancy

these presentations should trigger investigation, as maternal thrombophilia may be an underlying cause.

Staff and training implications

It is vital that only appropriately trained and competent staff should perform transabdominal and transvaginal early pregnancy scans. Sonographers, specialist nurses and clinicians should aspire to standardised ultrasound reports. Postgraduate trainees need supervision from their educational supervisor or lead clinician to ensure competency and observations of their skills in examination and scanning as part of their formative assessment of skills.

All recurrent miscarriage clinics should have a designated lead consultant with a special interest in recurrent miscarriage. In addition, all medical and nursing staff should undergo formal training in breaking bad news and training to provide emotional and psychological support.

Ideally, all gynaecologists should be able to conduct laparoscopic surgery in the management of ectopic pregnancy. Trainees should, in the future when these are available, complete an Advanced Training Skills Module in early pregnancy and laparoscopic surgery.

Opportunities for specialist training

There are training courses now available to specialist trainees as they progress through their careers. It is recommended that trainees complete the modules on intermediate ultrasound in gynaecology and intermediate ultrasound of early pregnancy complications before embarking on the Advanced Training Skills Module in Acute Gynaecology and Early Pregnancy.

Audit and research issues

As an essential component of clinical governance, all early pregnancy assessment units and recurrent miscarriage clinics should have regular meetings to review clinical guidelines and protocols. This would provide an ideal opportunity to discuss audits and to generate research ideas and discuss recruitment to national or international multicentre trials.

Regular audits should be undertaken to include patient choice regarding the management of miscarriage and ectopic pregnancy and complications associated with the various methods. Units should specifically include the medical and surgical management of ectopic pregnancy and the percentage of laparoscopic management of ectopic pregnancies, rates of ruptured ectopic pregnancies and incidence of failed diagnosis of ectopic pregnancy.

It is highly recommended that patient surveys with regard to patient satisfaction with facilities and counselling are included in order to identify areas that need improvement.

References

1. Association of Early Pregnancy Units. Early Pregnancy Information Centre [earlypregnancy.org.uk].
2. Royal College of Obstetricians and Gynaecologists. *Standards for Gynaecology.* London: RCOG Press; 2008. p. 14–19 [www.rcog.org.uk/womens-health/clinical-guidance/standards-gynaecology].
3. Royal College of Obstetricians and Gynaecologists. *The Management of Early Pregnancy Loss.* Green-top Guideline No. 25. London: RCOG; 2006 [www.rcog.org.uk/womens-health/clinical-guidance/management-early-pregnancy-loss-green-top-25].
4. British Association of Sexual Health and HIV. *2006 UK National Guideline for the Management of Genital Tract Infection with Chlamydia trachomatis* [www.bashh.org/documents/61/61.pdf].
5. Royal College of Obstetricians and Gynaecologists. *Early Miscarriage: Information for You.* London: RCOG; 2008 [www.rcog.org.uk/files/rcog-corp/uploaded-files/PIEarlyMiscarriage2008.pdf].
6. Trinder J, Brocklehurst P, Porter R, et al. Management of miscarriage: expectant, medical or surgical? Results of randomised controlled trial, miscarriage treatment (MIST trial). *BMJ* 2006;332:1235–40.
7. Ankum WM. Management of first-trimester miscarriage. *Br J Hosp Med* 2008;69:380–3.
8. Royal College of Obstetricians and Gynaecologists. *The Management of Tubal Pregnancy.* Green-top Guideline No. 21. London: RCOG; 2004 [www.rcog.org.uk/womens-health/clinical-guidance/management-tubal-pregnancy-21-may-2004].
9. Jauniaux E, Farquharson RG, Christiansen OB, Exalto N. Evidence-based guidelines for the investigation and medical treatment of women with recurrent miscarriage. *Hum Reprod* 2006;21:2216–22.
10. Royal College of Obstetricians and Gynaecologists. *The Investigation and Treatment of Couples with Recurrent Miscarriage.* Green-top Guideline No. 17. London: RCOG; 1998 [www.rcog.org.uk/womens-health/clinical-guidance/investigation-and-treatment-couples-recurrent-miscarriage-green-top-].

CHAPTER 3
Infertility

Mark Hamilton

Key points

✓ All patients with infertility problems should have prompt access to an integrated multidisciplinary service that provides efficient and accurate assessment of their clinical situation.

✓ Care should be individualised to meet the particular needs of those seeking help.

✓ Care should be reinforced by access to adequate information and appropriate counselling services.

✓ Patients should be supported in making informed choices about their care.

✓ The 18-week referral-to-treatment pathway is an opportunity for commissioners and providers to work together to improve services.

✓ The involvement of general practitioners in initial investigation is integral to achieving the 18-week target.

✓ Patients should receive consistent advice in primary, secondary and tertiary settings.

✓ Multiple pregnancies are a major issue of concern and, if the problem is to be adequately addressed, commissioners and providers need to work together in formulating contracts which include the use of cryopreserved embryos in the definition of a treatment cycle.

✓ Gamete donation and preimplantation genetic diagnosis services need to be considered in the context of a national service framework.

✓ Delivery of high-quality specialist services demands availability of personnel with special skills. All staff should have access to training to meet their needs.

✓ The numbers of subspecialists and special interest consultants are presently inadequate to meet service requirements.

✓ A rolling audit programme should be in place at all stages in the pathway of care for patients and should regularly assess clinic and laboratory standards.

✓ Engagement in research should be encouraged in all settings and specialist and subspecialist centres should engage with national trials initiatives.

Introduction

Fertility problems affect as many as one in seven couples in the UK. A common definition employed in describing infertility is the inability of a couple to conceive following 12–24 months of exposure to pregnancy. About 85% of couples having regular unprotected intercourse will have achieved conception by the time 1 year has elapsed and, by 2 years, this figure will have reached 92%.[1]

The year 2008 saw the 30th anniversary of the birth of the first baby conceived by in vitro fertilisation (IVF), an extraordinary achievement that heralded a new age in the evolution of infertility care. Before 1978, infertility practice was founded on an evidence base that was, at best, patchy. There were few conditions, with the notable exception of the use of drugs to induce ovulation, for which specific directed therapy was available. With the advent of IVF, the range of clinical situations for which targeted therapy could be offered expanded enormously. Indeed, in the present day, IVF is now integral to the care pathway for virtually all diagnostic scenarios in infertility.

An appreciation of the need for evidence to underpin practice has been accompanied by resolve to establish recognised standards for care provision for patients with infertility problems. This recognises the need to establish a grounded structure for service delivery, assessing competence and clinical performance and the provision of education within a multidisciplinary fertility service setting. The British Fertility Society (BFS) and the RCOG set out a care provision charter which encapsulates this philosophy.[2]

Infertility care provision charter

All patients with infertility problems should have prompt access to an integrated multidisciplinary service that provides efficient and accurate assessment of their clinical situation. This should lead to individualised management founded on evidence based principles of care. Care should be reinforced by access to adequate information and appropriate counselling services. At all times, the infertile should be treated with respect, and supported in making informed choices about their care and management.[2]

Clinical standards and national guidelines

The charter makes clear that patients should be at the centre of service design. Guidelines on infertility care derived from an RCOG initiative and translated into a National Institute for Health and Clinical Excellence (NICE) publication in 2004.[3] The guidelines encompassed initial assessment, diagnostic tests and interventions short of assisted reproduction techniques, including surgery, and, ultimately, the role of IVF and associated technologies. Patients' views were an integral part of guideline development, underpinned by recognition that a major frustration for service users was inconsistency in access to both simple and complex care across the country. For the first time, it seemed that infertility as a clinical problem was recognised as a real health issue by the UK Government. The aspiration, supported politically at the highest level, was for equitable delivery of NHS-based care. Similar initiatives had already taken place in Scotland.

As will be discussed below, progress has indeed been made, particularly in terms of access to IVF, although this falls far short of the recommendations of the Secretary of State for Health at the time.[4] That said, the use of the NICE guideline has been of use to providers in informing discussions with commissioners in determining service design and criteria for access to care.

Specific to licensed treatments, a collaborative approach involving the Human Fertilisation and Embryology Authority (HFEA), the regulator for the sector, and the professional bodies has seen the development of standards and guidelines which form the body of the Code of Practice, now in its seventh edition.[5] This important publication, against which licensed centres are inspected and accredited, has also been moderated in recent years by the European Union Tissues and Cells Directive.[6] Rigorous standards are now applied to organisational components of service infrastructure, embracing quality management in particular, with its associated demands on documentation, audit, resource management, validation of processes and equipment and risk management, among others. Clinics work in a culture which continuously evaluates performance and strives for improvement. Inspection of centres by the regulator has evolved into a rigorous but supportive exercise with patient needs a core element of assessment.

Service model for infertility

Review of the NICE guideline will take place in 2010. It is likely that this review will reinforce the principles incorporated in the original publication, particularly in the context of IVF access. NICE suggested that patients should be able to use all embryos, fresh and frozen, derived from three separate episodes of ovarian stimulation, egg retrieval and in vitro fertilisation. Social criteria, such as marital status, body mass index, smoking, that need to be met to access funded treatment were not stipulated but an age range of 23–39 years was recommended. The NHS contracts for only 30–35% of national activity and, despite NICE guidance, great variance on access to funded care continues to frustrate patients and providers.[4]

The incorporation of infertility as a care pathway subject to the same 18-week referral-to-treatment targets as other health issues has been a further indication of its recognition as mainstream medicine from a commissioning perspective.[7] To achieve targets as tight as this will require energy, imagination and commitment from commissioners and providers working in partnership.

Community-based services

Integration of services for the infertile encompassing a consistent, streamlined and informed approach to care is essential for many reasons.[3] Community-based services include opportunities for primary prevention of infertility, such as education about the risks of unsafe sexual practices and information on the decline of fertility associated with female age, particularly after 35 years. Public health education is also important, with respect to the need to take folic acid and lifestyle adjustments such as smoking, alcohol and weight. Dietary and smoking cessation advice should be made available. The support that the general practitioner can provide to the service is an essential component of the 18-week initiative where simple work-up will enable patients to begin first definitive treatment earlier. Thus, progesterone monitoring, rubella assessment, chlamydia screening and semen analysis should be performed in line with current guidelines before referral to the fertility clinic. It may be helpful for the local fertility clinic to employ dedicated liaison staff to assist with the referral process and guideline dissemination. In some instances, tubal assessment might be organised in primary care, although before committing to intrusive investigation it would be wise to have information on semen quality beforehand. This can be difficult where the male partner has a different GP from the woman but improved communication within primary care can resolve this issue. Bearing in mind the statutory requirement in offering licensed treatment to take account of the welfare of the potential child or existing children, it is essential that GPs give this some thought at this early stage to avoid difficulties in later management.

Referral

The need for onward referral to secondary care may be obvious, particularly where there is a history of menstrual irregularity or amenorrhoea, where there is pelvic infection or where semen results are abnormal. Consideration of prompt referral should also be made where the duration of infertility is more than 2 years, the woman is 35 years of age or more or there is a history of previous treatment for cancer or of bloodborne virus infection. Where screening tests for sexually transmitted infections are positive, the involvement of genitourinary services will be required.

Secondary care

The secondary care (specialist) setting should offer the infertile couple access to advice in a multidisciplinary infertility clinic. Typically, this will facilitate clarification and expansion of the primary care assessment, history and examination. Such a clinic will offer 5-day-a-week services during office hours and clinic cover to cater for those requiring weekend supervision. Access to more complex diagnostic tests or treatment would be available, including laparoscopy, with treatment of simple endometriosis if required, hysteroscopy, with treatment of simple lesions, advanced endocrinology, genetic analysis and qualitative semen analysis such as swim-up tests. Ovulation induction, at least to the level of clomifene, would be available, with access to ultrasound scanning 7 days a week. Subject to the skills and experience of attendant staff it may be possible for selective salpingography, tubal surgery, laparoscopic or open treatment of endometriosis or fibroids to be performed. Gonadotrophin ovulation induction could be offered but only where there is access to ultrasound and biochemistry services 7 days a week.

All patients should receive education relevant to diagnosis and management, with open explanation of expectant and interventional options, including success rates and risks of treatment. Verbal and written information in a range of languages should be available. In addition, it would be expected that access to counselling support, not only during assessment and treatment but also in the aftermath of care, would be facilitated.

Tertiary care

The general practitioner or secondary-level care provider may wish to engage directly with tertiary level (subspecialist) services, particularly if the woman is in her late 30s, the duration of infertility is more than 4 years, if there is a suspicion of low ovarian reserve (high early-follicular follicle-stimulating hormone and/or estradiol levels), if semen quality is very poor or there is a history of vasectomy, with or without reversal. Such a clinic will be an HFEA-licensed centre offering assisted conception services including IVF/intracytoplasmic sperm injection and, potentially, gamete donation services, surrogacy and preimplantation genetic diagnosis, although these latter may be delivered in a regional or supraregional provider setting.

Advanced diagnostic tests will be available in a tertiary care centre. These might include magnetic resonance imaging, selective salpingography, additional tests of ovarian reserve and advance sperm analysis. Surgical treatment of advanced endometriosis will be available, with the input of a colorectal surgeon as required, although, for complex cases, a regional service may be offered in a different centre.

The lead-in licensed centres will have statutory responsibilities in the role of Person Responsible, answerable to the regulator. Quality management dictates that the Person Responsible should ensure that all processes and procedures within the centre should be documented and undergo regular review. Key elements in personnel management (staffing numbers, job descriptions, initial and update training, competence assessment, continuing professional development, records and internal communication) should be in place. All equipment and materials should be subject to procurement, verification, validation and traceability procedures in accordance with the regulatory standards. The Person Responsible should coordinate key performance indicator monitoring for care periodically, as appropriate. This will include assessment of user satisfaction, monitoring and resolution of complaints, staff suggestions, internal audit, inter-centre comparisons and inter-laboratory quality assurance. In addition, identification, investigation, recording and notification of serious adverse events and reactions will be required.

Special issues

The present level of multiple pregnancies after assisted conception is currently a matter of concern to the regulator. Initiatives to encourage a reduction in twin rates after IVF without prejudicing overall chances of a live birth have been subject to debate in recent times. Guidelines from the BFS and the Association of Clinical Embryologists have been published.[8] Commissioners and providers need to work closely together to ensure that contracts for IVF services take account of the need to include the use of cryopreserved embryos in the definition of a cycle of treatment or the national target of reducing multiple rates to 10% as a maximum over the next 3 years to 2012 will not be achievable.

Availability of sperm donation treatment in the UK is variable and, in some regions, through lack of recruitment of donors, there are now long waiting lists or even withdrawal of services. An overhaul of the national framework of donor recruitment and service provision has been called for and a model akin to that of the National Blood Service may be a solution.[9]

Preimplantation genetic diagnostic services require care in planning relevant to the number of centres which should be resourced to meet a national need. The intimate relationship which the IVF services require with specialist genetic clinical and laboratory personnel is an important consideration. Furthermore, storage of gonadal tissue, for example, for young people with cancer or other conditions where medical or surgical intervention may result in sterility may also need to be organised on a regional basis.

Training needs

The delivery of high-quality specialist services demands the availability of personnel with special skills. Medical and nurse training in infertility has been enhanced through accreditation courses in the general management of infertility and assisted conception. These were developed by the BFS in close collaboration with the RCOG and the Royal College of Nursing and have been complemented by specific skill courses in embryo transfer and ultrasound in infertility.[10] Uptake of these courses has been high, indicative of their relevance to the service. Furthermore, the regulator in inspection has an interest in establishing documentary proof of competency in delivery of services and the format of training encompassing acquisition of knowledge and skills which are logged and verified by a designated trainer is helpful in quality assurance of training. Similar rigour is now applied to the postgraduate certificate in clinical embryology course for embryologists developed by the Association of Clinical Embryologists. The Association of Biomedical Andrologists is developing a similar formalised scheme for technical staff delivering andrology services.

Subspecialist training numbers have historically been difficult to predict but there is a continued need for output from national training programmes. The development of the Advanced Training Skills Modules (ATSMs) in infertility will facilitate the opportunity for regional planning for specialist services in appointing individuals with the necessary experience to provide for the population's need in fertility care at all levels of complexity.

The role of the Person Responsible is complex and legally important. Training for such a role has been a matter of concern to the regulator and to the BFS. Before an individual can take up position as a Person Responsible, it is required that they undergo a formal induction programme facilitated by the HFEA. This induction encompasses a distance learning programme exploring aspects of regulation and quality management. Complementary to this programme, the BFS has established its own training programme modelled in format on the infertility modules and specifically geared to prospective leads in infertility centres.[10] This training focuses on additional elements of service leadership, including human resource management, budget planning and contracting and other important areas.

Audit

As indicated above, quality management requires a continuous process of measurement, evaluation and improvement in the quality of services. Audit is integral to this and there are numerous examples of potential key performance indicators which could be examined:

- Infertility clinic:
  - patient satisfaction surveys of infertility unit service (such as information, waiting, staff courtesy, communication)
  - waiting times to new appointment
  - adherence to chlamydia and rubella screening protocols
  - percentage of patients with completed first-line investigations at GP
  - clomifene (anovulation) pregnancy rate
  - gonadotrophin (anovulation) pregnancy rate
  - ovulation induction multiple pregnancy rates.
- Andrology laboratory:
  - waiting time for routine semen analysis result
  - patients who do not attend as a percentage of appointments
  - average percentage of motile sperm recovery in intrauterine insemination treatment preparations
  - sperm survival rates after cryopreservation
  - assisted reproduction treatment
  - percentage of cycles initiated reaching egg recovery
  - average percentage of 2 pronucleate eggs for all patients/eggs inseminated in IVF
  - average percentage of cleavage of 2 pronucleate eggs
  - embryo cryopreservation rates
  - survival rate of cryopreserved embryos
  - clinical pregnancies/cycle initiated
  - multiple pregnancies as percentage of total pregnancies.

Research issues

It is important that senior staff within fertility centres cultivate an atmosphere that is supportive of research. The evidence base in reproductive medicine and infertility practice has been thin and the need for a more robust science base to underpin recommendations on clinical care for our patients is apparent. The National Reproductive Health Research Network is an important initiative and, within the fertility sector, a Reproductive Medicine Clinical Studies Group has now been established. Specialist infertility centres should be expected to engage with the group in supporting clinical trials and staff within centres should be encouraged to contribute locally, regionally and nationally to research where possible.

References

1. Evers JLH. Female subfertility. *Lancet* 2002;360:151–9.
2. British Fertility Society, Royal College of Obstetricians and Gynaecologists. *Standards in the Care of the Infertile*. BFS/RCOG Joint Document. December 2006 [www.fertility.org.uk/news/pressrelease/07_05-BFS-RCOG.html].
3. National Collaborating Centre for Women's and Children's Health. *Fertility: Assessment and Treatment for People with Fertility Problems*. London: RCOG Press; 2004.
4. Kennedy R, Kingsland C, Rutherford A, Hamilton M, Ledger W. Implementation of the NICE guideline: recommendations of the British Fertility Society for national criteria for NHS funding of assisted conception. *Hum Fertil* 2006;9:181–9.
5. Human Fertilisation and Embryology Authority. *Code of Practice*. 7th ed. London: HFEA; 2008 [www.hfea.gov.uk/codeofpractice].
6. Department of Health. EU Tissues and Cells Directive [http://www.dh.gov.uk/en/Publichealth/Scientificdevelopmentgeneticsandbioethics/Tissue/Tissuegeneralinformation/DH_4136920].
7. Department of Health. 18 week commissioning pathway – infertility 2008: assessment and treatment of couples with fertility problems [http://author.pathwaysforhealth.org/xpath2007/xeditor/publisher.asp?d_ref=E9D6A208FFA949C4B396192B33DFD611&d_name=&o_mode=0].
8. Cutting R, Morroll D, Roberts SA, Pickering S, Rutherford A, on behalf of the British Fertility Society and Association of Clinical Embryologists. Elective single embryo transfer: guidelines for practice. *Hum Fertil* 2008;11:131–46.
9. Hamilton M, Pacey A. Sperm donation in the UK. *BMJ* 2008;337:a2318 [DOI: 10.1136/bmj.a2318].
10. British Fertility Services. BFS approved training programmes leading to certification [www.fertility.org.uk/education/index.html].

Useful websites

Association of Clinical Embryologists: www.embryologists.org.uk
British Fertility Society: www.fertility.org.uk
Human Fertilisation and Embryology Authority: www.hfea.gov.uk

CHAPTER 4

Acute gynaecology

Edmond Edi-Osagie

Key points

✓ Every centre that delivers elective gynaecology care should provide access to acute gynaecology services.

✓ Acute gynaecology services should be accessible round the clock and within 24 hours of referral.

✓ Units should consider combining acute gynaecology and early pregnancy into emergency gynaecology services.

✓ Every acute gynaecology unit should have a lead consultant responsible for that service.

✓ Units should adopt and publish a care pathway that reflects local circumstances.

✓ Evidence-based protocols and guidelines for common conditions should be available.

✓ Units should have a robust system for review and handover of outpatients and inpatients.

✓ Every unit should have access to training programmes for medical and nursing staff.

✓ There should be a rolling audit programme that feeds into clinical governance structures.

✓ Units should ensure a robust risk management and clinical governance system.

Introduction

Emergency gynaecology is rapidly developing in the UK but remains mostly fragmented into early pregnancy and acute gynaecology. Early pregnancy units provide care to women in the first 20 weeks of pregnancy while acute gynaecology units deliver care to women who are not pregnant. Conditions treated include pelvic inflammatory disease, acute pelvic pain, lower genital tract infections, excessive vaginal bleeding, acute pelvic mass complications, vulval abscesses, genital tract injuries (including those resulting from sexual assault), acute urinary retention and ovarian hyperstimulation syndrome (OHSS). Emergency contraception is also provided in such units.

There is a dearth of literature on patient and service surveys, treatment guidelines and protocols and standards for acute gynaecology. A nationwide audit was therefore commissioned for this work, to facilitate understanding of the state of acute gynaecology services in the UK. Much of the other material for this chapter was limited but useful in establishing a foundation for the development of acute gynaecology.

The service user's view

There is a dearth of evidence for acute gynaecology and a comprehensive search yielded no patient or service surveys. Seventy-six responses were received from a nationwide audit of acute gynaecology units.[1] Results show that:

- 33 centres (44%) had early pregnancy units and provided acute gynaecology from wards (n = 14, 42%) or shared premises including accident and emergency (n = 10, 30%). Nine (27%) centres had no provision for acute gynaecology and, of these, six (67%) had no consultant lead.
- 19 centres (25%) had separate early pregnancy units and acute gynaecology units. Four (21%) delivered acute gynaecology from dedicated premises; three (16%) from shared premises and 19 (63%) from ward-based units. Six (32%) opened for restricted hours all week while 13 (68%) opened round-the-clock.
- 21 centres (28%) had combined early pregnancy and acute gynaecology units. Seventeen (81%) were delivered from dedicated premises while four (19%) were ward-based. Eight (38%) opened for restricted hours all week, 12 (57%) had restricted weekday opening and one (5%) opened round-the-clock.
- The status of three centres (4%) was unclear, as they claimed to deliver only acute gynaecology but also responded to questions about early pregnancy.

- 66 of 67 centres (99%) delivering (99%) accepted general practitioner referrals, 20 (30%) self-referrals, 18 (27%) walk-ins and 44 (66%) other department referrals.
- 21 centres (31%) used appointment systems for new referrals and 40 (60%) did same for follow-up visits.
- 11 centres (16%) had ultrasound machines on the units; 16 (24%) used dedicated scan slots; 14 (21%) had a machine and a sonographer on the units while 24 (36%) had no scanning service. Forty-one centres (61%) relied on sonographers for scans, seven (10%) relied on consultants, six (9%) used staff grades/specialist registrars and three (4%) used nurse sonographers.
- 18 centres (27%) had access to dedicated daytime emergency theatre lists, six (9%) used slots on elective lists, 22 (33%) used National Confidential Enquiry into Patient Outcome and Death lists and 17 (25%) out-of-hours emergency lists.
- 38 centres (50%) provided training for senior house officers, 41 (54%) for specialist registrars and 30 (39%) for nurses.
- 58 centres (76%) had consultant leads. The service was consultant-led in another 26 (39%), specialist registrar or staff grade-led in 19 (28%), senior house officer-led in eight (12%) and nurse-led in 10 (15%).

Clinical standards and national guidelines

It is practical to address the issues of clinical standards and national guidelines separately.

Clinical standards

Two recent RCOG publications addressed gynaecology standards. *Standards for Gynaecology* included standards for pelvic inflammatory disease.[2] *Gynaecology Emergency Services Standards of Practice and Service Organisation* addressed emergency gynaecology standards.[3]

Service model
Units delivering gynaecological care should provide access to acute gynaecology as a separate service or combined with early pregnancy. Size, case mix and available manpower should influence the decision on separate or combined units. Combined units offer many advantages,

including efficient use of limited medical, nursing, midwifery and sonography resources and dual use of premises and theatre slots.

Location of units

Whether units are located on the site of elective gynaecology centres should be determined by size, case mix, available manpower and geography. Small centres that are geographically closely located should consider shared units, locating these on one hospital or community site and developing robust pathways for patient transfers and access to support services.

Premises

Acute gynaecology units should ideally be located in dedicated premises that ensure ease of access, privacy and confidentiality and access to support services. Units combining acute gynaecology and early pregnancy would find these objectives easier to achieve. Shared premises are acceptable alternatives, especially in small centres, but locating acute gynaecology services on inpatient wards is not ideal.

Opening times

Acute gynaecology services should provide round-the-clock access, as well as access within 24 hours of referral. Centres should consider innovative ways of achieving these goals, including collaborations with neighbouring units for out-of-hours work. It is unacceptable for acute gynaecology services to be inaccessible for any length of time.

Support services

There should be ready access to laboratory services (haematology, biochemistry and endocrinology), ultrasound and radiology (magnetic resonance imaging and computed tomography) and these should be accessible out-of-hours. Units should consider innovative ways of ensuring the availability of ultrasound, the value of which has been well demonstrated in such settings.[4] There should be access to high dependency and intensive care facilities, preferably on the same site. Alternatively, shared care pathways should be developed with centres where they are located.

Theatre access

There should be ready theatre access to avoid delays and prevent queues for theatre. This calls for innovative approaches, including 'outpatient surgery' for minor conditions using established protocols.[5] Out-of-hours surgery should be discouraged, except when absolutely unavoidable. Acceptable alternatives include 'ring-fencing' entire lists and 'ring-fencing' slots on elective lists (numbers and frequency to be determined by need).

Health records management

Units should consider innovative ways of ensuring that patient records are accessible to other healthcare providers. Handheld records should be implemented locally and serious consideration should be given to electronic record systems that would also facilitate the collation of data for audit, research and submission to regulatory agencies and link up to future NHS systems.

Guidelines for practice

Units should develop local protocols and policies based on nationally agreed guidelines where these are available. The RCOG Green-top Guideline, *Management of Acute Pelvic Inflammatory Disease*, should be adapted for local use.[6] Guidelines for managing lower genital tract infections can be adapted from those provided by the British Association of Sexual Health and HIV.[7] National Institute for Health and Clinical Excellence guidelines for heavy menstrual bleeding can be adapted for managing excessive vaginal bleeding.[8] Units should adapt the RCOG Green-top Guideline on *Management of Ovarian Hyperstimulation Syndrome* for local use.[9] Useful guidance for managing acute pelvic mass complications can be obtained from a number of recent reviews.[10] Guidance for managing acute pelvic pain can be obtained from the Pelvic Pain Support Network.[11] Emergency contraception guidelines can be adapted from those of the Faculty of Sexual and Reproductive Health Care.[12]

Patient focus

Patient information leaflets should be available in all clinical areas and should detail the processes of care and should also include unit telephone numbers. Patients groups should be involved in the development of such leaflets to ensure more relevant, readable and understandable material. Units with large non-English speaking populations should interpret the material into major local languages. Generic patient information for pelvic inflammatory disease and OHSS is available from the RCOG.[13,14]

Service model and care pathways

Figure 4.1 details a prototype acute gynaecology care pathway which units can adapt for local use.

Referral patterns

Units should determine and publish widely their referral base and acceptance criteria. Referral patterns should be carefully considered to ensure balance between obligations of an emergency service and quality of care. Telephone triage should be considered within the referral process, as this reduces medical workload and cost in comparable settings.[15] Smaller centres should have shared care pathways with larger centres for patients requiring access to specialist, tertiary or intensive care.

Process

Units should develop triage systems for new cases using modified early warning scores (MEWS) for prompt and accurate assessment and feeding into traffic-light trigger systems for prioritising cases. Senior nurses should undertake triage to enhance formulation of MEWS-based action plans.

NHS Direct in England and Wales and NHS 24 in Scotland are designed to offer both in-hours and out-of-hours triage services to help manage the workload in general practice, as well as direct advice to patients and there needs to be continuing engagement with these institutions to establish agreed care standards and pathways and to quality assure the acute gynaecological patient process. At the very minimum, advice given via these sources should reflect practice within the local acute gynaecological unit.

Full prioritised clinical assessments should follow triage and should lead to care plans that involve relevant professionals. Operational policies for escalating cases up to consultant level should be developed. Protocols and guidelines should detail criteria for outpatient and inpatient medical and surgical care, expected length of inpatient stay, involvement of other professionals and follow-up arrangements.

There should be regular reviews of difficult or challenging cases by senior clinicians (including consultant and specialist nurse). An approach to achieving this in outpatient settings is daily record reviews at

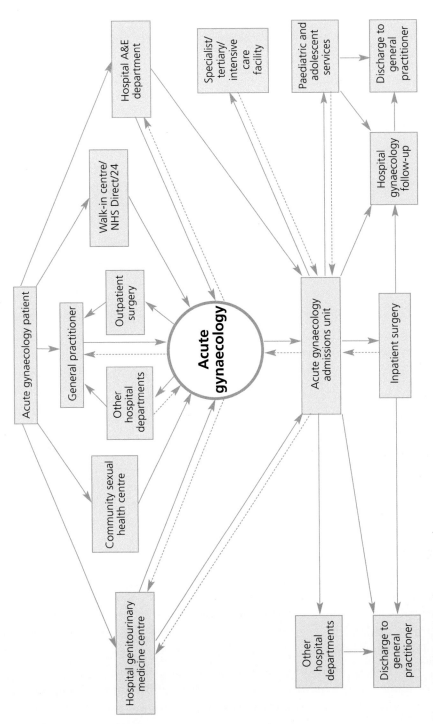

Figure 4.1 Acute gynaecology care pathway

consultant-led emergency ward rounds (including weekends). Acute gynaecology inpatients should be reviewed at these ward rounds at least daily and within 24 hours of admission. There should be formal face-to-face handovers of care between changing shifts of doctors and nurses or telephone handovers when circumstances warrant.

Special issues

Innovative and efficient ways of managing follow-up appointments should be explored to avoid overburdening systems and compromising acute care. Consideration should be given to appointment or clinic systems and telephone follow-up in the light of its proven benefits.[15]

A comprehensive governance structure should be in place, with robust systems for identification and reporting of risk and investigation of clinical incidents, including clinical reviews and root cause analysis where appropriate, implementation of action plans and feedback mechanisms to continually update staff on outcomes.

Medical staffing

Units should have acute gynaecology on-call rotas with consultants freed up from elective work commitments. The rota should ideally be separate from the obstetric rota, ensuring that a consultant is available for acute gynaecology at all times and this should be immediately achievable in large units (over 4000 deliveries) which have sufficient consultant numbers.[16] Units with fewer than eight consultants will find this difficult without consultant expansion and should consider a combined rota for obstetrics and gynaecology with middle-grade support.

Staff and training needs

Several factors should influence the make-up of clinical teams, including whether units are stand-alone or combined, size, case mix, opening times and referral patterns. There should be a suitably qualified consultant lead with responsibility for clinical organisation, setting and maintaining standards and governance. This responsibility should be adequately reflected in the job plan.[3]

Units should be staffed by multidisciplinary teams that include specialist nurses, healthcare support workers and administrative staff, with local determination of numbers and ratios. Large units and those dealing with complex or specialist cases will need middle-grade medical staff and this should be built into on-call rotas. Doctors in training require exposure to acute gynaecology to fulfil important training needs but the era of staffing units with trainees who are left to fend for themselves is long gone. Trust-grade doctors and clinical fellows previously provided a ready source of trained middle-grade manpower but it is now difficult to recruit to these posts. Evidence suggests that there are no appreciable differences between care delivered by doctors and by well-trained nurses in health outcomes for patients, processes of care, resource use or cost in primary care settings.[17] Units may wish to also explore the option of training and using advanced nurse practitioners.

Staff training should be a priority, irrespective of who provides care. Core staff should have knowledge of sexual health and should be duly certified where necessary. Regular educational and governance meetings should take place in units with involvement of other key personnel in the obstetrics and gynaecology team, counsellors, anaesthetists, theatre practitioners, general practitioners, genitourinary medicine specialists and laboratory personnel. Timing and frequency of these meetings should be guided by size and stage of development. New units need frequent interdisciplinary and review meetings, while fully established units with well-developed and integrated care pathways might focus more on clinical and governance meetings. Units should strive to include acute gynaecology as regular features in clinical meetings, which should be held at least monthly and should link into clinical governance arrangements.

Opportunities for specialist training

There should be in-house training programmes for both medical and nursing staff or collaborations with neighbouring units to provide same. Specialty training committees should work to designate certain units within each deanery as providers of advanced training towards the acute gynaecology and early pregnancy Advanced Training Skills Module. Unit training programmes in obstetrics and gynaecology and general practice should include sessions on genitourinary medicine.

Resource implications

There are obvious resource implications of these recommendations, which should be balanced against quality-of-care improvements that should accrue. The recommendations should potentially curtail adverse clinical events and litigation. Efficiency cost savings would release spare capacity and potentially lead to increased income from payment by results. Unit directors should work to develop business plans reflecting these issues for consideration by their corporate teams.

Audit and research issues

There should be a rolling programme of audit of clinical processes and outcomes determined by both local and national priorities. Units should regularly audit compliance with local protocols and guidelines and with relevant national guidelines that are adoptable locally, such as RCOG Green-top Guidelines on management of acute pelvic inflammatory disease and OHSS.[8,9] Research should be actively encouraged within individual units and as part of collaborative multicentre initiatives. There is a dearth of evidence in acute gynaecology and research efforts should focus particularly on qualitative issues and the role of inpatient and outpatient surgical interventions.

References

1. Wan L, Edi-Osagie ECO. New directions in the provision of acute gynaecology services for non-pregnant women in the UK. Personal communication.
2. Royal College of Obstetricians and Gynaecologists. *Standards for Gynaecology: Report of a Working Party*. London: RCOG Press; 2008 [www.rcog.org.uk/womens-health/clinical-guidance/standards-gynaecology].
3. Royal College of Obstetricians and Gynaecologists. *Gynaecology: Emergency Services Standards of Practice and Service Organisation*. Good Practice No 9. London: RCOG; 2009 [www.rcog.org.uk/good-practice-gynaecology-emergency-services].
4. Haider Z, Condous G, Khalid A, Kirk E, Mukri F, Van Calster B, *et al*. Impact of the availability of sonography in the acute gynaecology unit. *Ultrasound Obstet Gynecol* 2006;28:207–13.
5. Ferry J, Rankin L. Low cost, patient acceptable, local analgesia approach to gynaecological outpatient surgery: a review of 817 consecutive procedures. *Aust N Z J Obstet Gynaecol* 2008;34:453–56.
6. Royal College of Obstetricians and Gynaecologists. *Management of Acute Pelvic Inflammatory Disease*. Green-top Guideline No. 32. London: RCOG; 2008 [www.rcog.org.uk/womens-health/clinical-guidance/management-acute-pelvic-inflammatory-disease-32].

7. British Association of Sexual Health and HIV. Guidelines. BASHH Clinical Effectiveness Group guidelines. [www.bashh.org/guidelines].

8. National Institute for Health and Clinical Excellence. *Heavy Menstrual Bleeding*. London: NICE; 2007 [www.nice.org.uk/Guidance/CG44].

9. Royal College of Obstetricians and Gynaecologists. *Management of Ovarian Hyperstimulation Syndrome*. Green-top Guideline No. 5. London: RCOG; 2006 [www.rcog.org.uk/womens-health/clinical-guidance/management-ovarian-hyperstimulation-syndrome-green-top-5].

10. McWilliams GD, Hill MJ, Dietrich CS 3rd. Gynecologic emergencies. *Surg Clin North Am* 2008;88:265–83.

11. Pelvic Pain Support Network. Guidelines [www.pelvicpain.org.uk/ci-guidelines.php].

12. Faculty of Family Planning and Reproductive Health Care Clinical Effectiveness Unit. FFPRHC Guidance (April 2006) Emergency contraception. *J Fam Plan Reprod Health Care* 2006;32:121–8 [www.ffprhc.org.uk/admin/uploads/449_Emergency ContraceptionCEUguidance.pdf].

13. Royal College of Obstetricians and Gynaecologists. *Acute Pelvic Inflammatory Disease (PID): What the RCOG Guideline Means for You*. London: RCOG; 2004 [www.rcog.org.uk/womens-health/clinical-guidance/acute-pelvic-inflammatory-disease-pid].

14. Royal College of Obstetricians and Gynaecologists. *Ovarian Hyperstimulation Syndrome: What You Need to Know*. London: RCOG; 2007 [www.rcog.org.uk/womens-health/clinical-guidance/ovarian-hyperstimulation-syndrome-what-you-need-know].

15. Leibowitz R, Day S, Dunt D. A systematic review of the effect of different models of after-hours primary medical care services on clinical outcomes, medical workload, and patient and GP satisfaction. *Fam Pract* 2003;20:311–17.

16. Royal College of Obstetricians and Gynaecologists. *The Future Role of the Consultant: A Working Party Report*. London: RCOG Press; 2005 [www.rcog.org.uk/womens-health/clinical-guidance/future-role-consultant].

17. Laurant M, Reeves D, Hermens R, Braspenning J, Grol R, Sibbald B. Substitution of doctors by nurses in primary care. *Cochrane Database Syst Rev* 2005;18(2):CD001271.

CHAPTER 5

Sexual and reproductive health services

Alison Bigrigg, Audrey Brown and Kay Mcallister

Key points

✓ Sexual and reproductive healthcare services are client focused, encompassing the diverse needs of the population.

✓ Comprehensive information about local sexual healthcare services needs to be available in both the public and professional domains.

✓ Sexual and reproductive healthcare provision is based on evidence-based guidance and standards from a range of relevant professional bodies.

✓ All staff providing sexual health care should be aware of and have appropriate training in the relevant standards.

✓ Staff should be aware of and use appropriate care pathways to ensure effective and efficient health care.

✓ Multi-agency partnership working supports sexual and reproductive healthcare services to provide a holistic care model.

✓ Obstetricians and gynaecologists require skills and knowledge in sexual and reproductive health practice and this can be achieved through DFSRH.

✓ Specialist sexual and reproductive healthcare services should be led by a consultant with appropriate training in sexual and reproductive health.

✓ Investment in sexual and reproductive health services is cost effective for the NHS.

✓ Incorporating audit and research into sexual and reproductive healthcare practice is essential to further improve sexual and reproductive health outcomes, at both individual and population levels.

Introduction

Sexual health service users expect a choice of free, confidential, non-judgmental services provided by trained staff to nationally recognised standards. They expect information to be consistent, accurate and up to date. This was the advice given to Quality Improvement Scotland (QIS) in 2008 by an advocacy group comprising 17 different voluntary organisations.[1]

Men and women seeking sexual health information, advice and treatment are generally well. However, they may find it embarrassing to talk openly with a professional about sex. It is therefore especially important in these consultations to:

- avoid stereotyping
- avoid appearing critical or judgmental (foolish, feckless, promiscuous, too young, should know better)
- to listen and understand, not interrogate
- give enough time and information (the reasons behind and options for women requesting the pill or a pregnancy test need to be sympathetically explored rather than simply complied with)
- to give encouragement to voice fears and anxieties, including issues around alcohol and violence.

At a service level, evidence shows a need to empower people to have confidence, personal control and choice in managing their sexual health care and service use.[2] To enable them to do this, information must be provided on:

- what, where and when services are available
- how to access services
- who they will see and how they will be treated
- confidentiality of the service
- the choices they will have
- whether they can bring anyone with them.

Clinical standards and national guidelines

Appropriate standards and nationally accepted guidelines are fundamental to the provision of any specialist service. Sexual and reproductive health services have been influenced for many years by several bodies, including:

- the Faculty of Sexual and Reproductive Healthcare of the RCOG (FSRH)
- the Royal College of Obstetricians and Gynaecologists
- the British Association for Sexual Health and HIV (BASHH)
- the National Institute for Health and Clinical Excellence (NICE)
- the Scottish Intercollegiate Guidelines Network (SIGN)
- Quality Improvement Scotland.

The publication of guidelines at a national level aids the clinician both at a commissioning or service level and with individual cases at the clinical level. Politics surrounding sexual and reproductive health provision vary between the countries of the UK and within countries at health board level, depending on whether services are based in primary or secondary care. These differences can have huge resource implications for service provision. However, publication of clinical standards helps to support clinicians in the provision of high-quality care to clients.

An obvious example of a standard which has resulted in improved care for women is the NICE publication on long-acting reversible contraception (LARC).[3] This document has led to a concerted effort by general practitioners, sexual and reproductive healthcare doctors and hospital-based gynaecologists to change practice and to allow an increased uptake of LARCs. This change has involved improved training and education of both medical and nursing staff, aided by other guidelines such as the contraceptive guidelines from the clinical effectiveness unit of FSRH and the UK adaptation of the World Health Organization *Medical Eligibility Criteria for Contraceptive Use*.[4] Overall, the uptake of LARC methods has increased, associated with a national reduction in the proportion of women undergoing sterilisation procedures.

More importantly, there has been a move over the past few years for joint working between FSRH, RCOG and BASHH. The continuation of this trend will enable joint national guidelines and standards to be published. It is envisaged that, with more community-based sexual and reproductive health care being provided in integrated settings, joint guidelines will provide the framework for continued high-quality care. This will benefit both women and men seeking help and advice.

Service model

The 10-year National Strategy for Sexual Health and HIV clearly lays out a plan for service delivery (Figure 5.1).[5] Level 1 services should be available within general practice and include testing for female sexually transmitted infections, HIV counselling and testing and contraceptive information. Level 2 services may be provided within primary care teams with a special interest in sexual health, or by other service providers such as obstetrics and gynaecology departments. This service level includes insertion of intrauterine contraceptive devices, testing for male sexually transmitted infections and partner notification.

Level 3

specialist SRH care units

highly specialised contraception • HIV care • infection management
clinical governance support to level 1 and 2 providers

Level 2 services

primary care team with special interest in SRH/O&G department

IUCD insertion • male STI testing • partner notification

Level 1 services

general practice

female STI testing • HIV counselling/testing • contraceptive information

---

Figure 5.1 Sexual and reproductive service outline

Specialist sexual and reproductive healthcare units are expected to provide level 3 services, including highly specialised contraception, HIV care and infection management. These services will also provide clinical and governance support to level 1 and 2 providers.

Implementation of this sexual health strategy has led to changes in the skill mix of staff, with the introduction of more patient group directions and nurse prescribers. Similarly, managed clinical networks will be of increasing benefit, particularly if multidisciplinary working, including user groups and the voluntary sector, is further developed.

Service provision

Sexual and reproductive health care is different from most other specialties. In general, clients are young, healthy and symptom-free. Most consultations are initiated from a self-referral basis and so services in their various forms are a major factor in influencing attendance. Information needs to be directed as much towards the public as to other healthcare professionals. Models of services need to be considered from several aspects:

- equity of service provision
- equity of client access
- type of service provided.

Equity of service provision is often difficult to achieve throughout any country. This is more so when comparing urban with rural areas, where access can be challenging. All services need to take into account the difficulties of clients in rural areas. These range from transport to services, less availability and choice of services and possible less anonymity in smaller communities.

Equity of client access must take into account many client characteristics. These include age, ethnicity, reasons for attendance and social status. Central to this is an understanding of the client base within the locality of the service. Provision of specific services for young people is known to increase their uptake. Similarly, establishing services for ethnic minorities within the communities where people live leads to better uptake. This can be enhanced by simple measures such as leaflets and posters advertising the service printed in different languages. There are long-established inequalities to access within all areas of health care, such as homelessness, learning disabilities and poor socio-economic status. It is imperative that any proposed service takes into account these groups and provides suitably tailored services. This may be a specialised clinic with support workers, carers or health visitors or a service with a domiciliary or outreach element.

Types of service

Sexual and reproductive health services have evolved over time, with changes relating to timing and style as well as content of services. There is probably no one timing and style which suits all services and the client base will influence this. For example, some client groups prefer the availability of a drop-in service and others, perhaps with a work or study schedule, would prefer a fixed appointment time. Similarly, evening, early morning, lunchtime and Saturday opening times are more important for working clients and daytime may be more acceptable for those with school-age children.

In many parts of the UK, sexual and reproductive health services are co-located with genitourinary medicine services but few centres offer a truly integrated service. The provision of an integrated service has many advantages for clients, where clinical care often overlaps.

Any service provision must take into account the needs, wishes and preferences of the client base, including the provision of appropriate information in a style and content that is understandable to the client.

■ Care pathways

Irrespective of the size, site and timing of services, it is imperative that clearly defined care pathways are in place. These pathways include the links from general practitioners in primary care to sexual and reproductive health services and from these services to acute and tertiary care. These links with general practitioners are particularly useful when combined efforts are required for national targets such as partner notification, LARC provision and chlamydia screening. Similarly, the link between sexual and reproductive health care services and acute and tertiary care needs to be robust if the appropriate onward referral of clients is to be effected. In some clinical situations, these care pathways are part of everyday practice, ensuring seamless transition of care (for example for those seeking termination of pregnancy or female sterilisation).[6,7]

Sexual and reproductive health services are also often involved in multi-agency working, including the voluntary sector. All staff should be made aware of and have access to clearly written protocols and guidelines regarding the correct pathway of care for clients.

Staff and training needs

Provision of a competent and comprehensive sexual and reproductive health service requires an appropriate staffing capacity, equipped with the skills to deliver care of the highest standard. The FSRH has brought together recommendations from the sexual health strategies for England and Scotland and the Medical Foundation for AIDS and Sexual Health standards, and has published services standards for sexual health services.[8] These standards recognised that, as a minimum, sexual and reproductive health services should be consultant led, with one whole-time equivalent consultant for each 125,000 of population. This is mirrored in the NHS QIS Standards for Sexual Health Services, which again identify the essential criteria of appropriate service leadership, by a consultant with subspecialty training in sexual and reproductive health. An RCOG workforce planning review in Scotland acknowledged that there is currently a shortage of sexual and reproductive health consultants in post and that subspecialty training slots are required, to meet the projected consultant workforce needs of the future.[9]

Consultants leading sexual and reproductive health services are supported in delivery of the service by a wide range of other staff, including staff-grade and associate specialists, sexual health nursing staff, pharmacists and youth workers. It is essential that all staff working in sexual and reproductive health have appropriate training and are able to meet continuing educational needs. As a minimum, doctors working in sexual and reproductive health should have achieved the Diploma of the FSRH, a competence-based qualification. Doctors providing additional contraceptive services, such as insertion of intrauterine contraceptive devices or subdermal contraceptive implants, can obtain a letter of competence in these techniques. Reaccreditation of the FSRH qualifications requires evidence of continuing professional development and demonstration of continued practice of the skill.

Nurses working in sexual and reproductive health services should have a recognised postgraduate qualification in sexual health and, again, require support to ensure continuing professional education and training.

It is recognised that staff working across the range of obstetrics and gynaecology services will deliver aspects of sexual and reproductive health care as an integral part of the care provided; for example, provision of contraception following termination of pregnancy or testing for *Chlamydia trachomatis* in an infertility clinic. It is essential that acute service staff are appropriately trained to provide this care, for example by obtaining and maintaining the DFSRH or equivalent. In addition, staff are likely to deal with a variety of complex clinical scenarios and should receive appropriate training and support in confidentiality and child protection.

Opportunities for specialist training

All staff working in obstetrics and gynaecology will require knowledge and skills in sexual and reproductive health care; the specialty training logbook includes a module on sexual and reproductive health. However, some trainees may wish to gain a more in-depth knowledge and experience, in the advanced training years, and can undertake the Advanced Training Skills Module (ATSM) in Sexual Health. It is likely that a major part of this module would be undertaken in the community setting. This might be combined with an ATSM, for example, in menopause or abortion care, for a trainee looking develop a special interest in sexual and reproductive health.[10,11,12]

It is expected that a separate Certificate of Completion of Training for sexual and reproductive health will be in place around 2010.

Resource implications

It is well established that 'family planning services are highly cost effective and provide a high rate of return for the NHS'.[13] The National Strategy for Sexual Health and HIV estimated the prevention of unplanned pregnancy saves the NHS over £2.5billion a year. It also stated that the monetary value of preventing a single onward transmission of HIV to be £0.5–1.0million in terms of individual health benefits, treatment and care. Despite this economic evidence, it remains a struggle for individual services to convince commissioners of the importance of funding community-based services. In the past 10 years, however, the previously 'Cinderella' services of sexual and reproductive health have emerged as an essential element of the NHS Health Improvement Programme. This has coincided with the provision of a consultant-led service.

Despite the overwhelming economic case for sexual and reproductive health services, it is essential to ensure that services are provided in the most cost-efficient and effective manner. This includes reviewing factors, such as type of service (walk-in or appointment), new to return visit ratio and staff skill mix. Adopting modern technology is also crucial, for example, providing results to patients by telephone or texting services.

Research and guidelines should attempt to assess cost effectiveness of their proposals. The NICE guidance on LARC included a full economic analysis, which showed the use of long-acting methods was more cost effective than user-dependent methods, even if only used for 1 year. This greatly enhanced the impact of the guideline in changing practice.

Audit and research issues

Despite the availability of contraception and sexually transmitted infection treatment free at the point of delivery for many decades, the UK has among the highest teenage birth rates in Western Europe, rising sexually transmitted infection rates and increasingly risky sexual behaviours. There is an urgent need for research to understand why this should be and to explore health, educational and cultural methods of influencing sexual health and increasing the effectiveness of health interventions. Unfortunately, in recent years, research activity has tended to focus on commercial pharmaceutical studies.

As the specialty of sexual and reproductive health emerges in the 21st century, it is expected and hoped that research and audit in the area will develop and positively influence service delivery and outcomes. Research is required at an individual consultation level, service level and population basis.

When guidelines are published, suggestions for audit and research to explore issues where there is little evidence should be included. The FSRH has indicated it will shortly produce a research and audit strategy, a development which will be most welcome.

References

1. National Health Service Quality Improvement Scotland. *Sexual Health Services: Standards.* Edinburgh: NHS QIS; 2008 [www.nhshealthquality.org./nhsqis/4138.html].
2. Medical Foundation for AIDS and Sexual Health. *Recommended Standards for Sexual Health Services.* London: MedFash; 2005 [www.medfash.org.uk/publications/current.html].
3. National Collaborating Centre for Women's and Children's Health. *Long-acting Reversible Contraception: The Effective and Appropriate Use of Long-acting Reversible Contraception.* Clinical Guideline. London: RCOG Press; 2005 [guidance.nice.org.uk/CG30].

4. Faculty of Family Planning and Reproductive Healthcare. *UK Medical Eligibility Criteria for Contraceptive Use (UKMEC 2005/2006)*. London: FFPRC; 2006 [www.ffprhc.org.uk/].

5. Department of Health. *The National Strategy for Sexual Health and HIV*. London: DH; 2000 [www.dh.gov.uk/en/Consultations/Closedconsultations/DH_4084674].

6. Royal College of Obstetricians and Gynaecologists. *The Care of Women Requesting Induced Abortion*. Evidence-based Clinical Guideline No. 7. London: RCOG Press; 2004.

7. Royal College of Obstetricians and Gynaecologists. *Male and Female Sterilisation*. Evidence-based Clinical Guideline No. 4. London: RCOG Press; 2004.

8. Faculty of Family Planning and Reproductive Health Care. *Service Standards for Sexual Health Services*. London: FFPRC; 2006 [www.ffprhc.org.uk].

9. Royal College of Obstetricians and Gynaecologists. *The Future of Obstetrics and Gynaecology in Scotland: Service Provision and Workforce Planning*. London: RCOG Press; 2005 [www.rcog.org.uk/womens-health/clinical-guidance/future-obstetrics-and-gynaecology-scotland].

10. Royal College of Obstetricians and Gynaecologists. ATSM Sexual Health Advanced Training Skills. 2008 [www.rcog.org.uk/curriculum-module/atsm-sexual-health].

11. Royal College of Obstetricians and Gynaecologists. ATSM Menopause Advanced Training Skills. 2008 [www.rcog.org.uk/curriculum-module/atsm-menopause].

12. Royal College of Obstetricians and Gynaecologists. ATSM Abortion Care Advanced Training Skills. 2008 [www.rcog.org.uk/curriculum-module/atsm-abortion-care-0].

13. NHS Centre for Reviews and Dissemination, University of York. Preventing and reducing the adverse effects of unintended teenage pregnancies. *Effective Health Care Bull* 1997;3(1):1–12.

CHAPTER 6
Termination of pregnancy

Kamal Ojha and Arti Matah

Key points

✓ Services for termination of pregnancy should be offered as part of comprehensive reproductive health care.

✓ All termination of pregnancy care facilities should offer contraception services or referral to such services.

✓ Protocols on post-procedure contraception should be developed and a supply of contraceptives should be available at facilities for termination of pregnancy.

✓ Counselling and support services should be commissioned as part of the package of care.

Introduction

Termination of pregnancy is one of the most commonly performed gynaecological procedures in Great Britain. At least one-third of British women will have had an abortion by the time they reach the age of 45 years. In 2007, for women resident in England and Wales:[1]

- the total number of terminations was 198,500, compared with 193,700 in 2006, a rise of 2.5%
- the rate among girls under 16 years of age was 4.4/1000 and that in the under-18 age group, 19.8/1000, both rates higher than in 2006
- 90% of terminations were carried out before 13 weeks of gestation; 70% at under 10 weeks
- medical terminations accounted for 35% of the total, compared with 30% in 2006.

The RCOG, in 2004, published national evidence-based guidelines on *The Care of Women Requesting Abortion*, which set quality standards for abortion services.[2]

The aim of a termination of pregnancy service is to provide high-quality, efficient, effective, and legal and comprehensive care, which respects the dignity, individuality and rights of women to exercise personal choice over their treatment. Ideally, this service should be an integral component of a broader service for reproductive and sexual health, encompassing contraception and management of sexually transmitted infections. The objective should be to offer impartial support and advice to all women with an unintended pregnancy, who request a termination, regardless of age, ethnicity, language, disability, religious or personal circumstances.

The service user's view

Management of termination services should be prioritised to reflect what women want: particularly decreased waiting times for terminations and greater ease and convenience in booking appointments.

Clinical standards and national guidelines

Access and referral to termination of pregnancy services

Any woman considering termination of pregnancy should have access to clinical assessment. Termination services should have local strategies in place for providing information to both women and healthcare professionals on the choices available within the service and on routes of access to the service. Prompt referral from primary care should be monitored and a central booking service for direct or onward referral, with clear clinical care pathways, should be in place in all services. All possible referrers should be made aware of the RCOG recommendations concerning the time limits on referral for termination and procedures. Improved information on access to termination services should be clearly signposted in all general practices and other primary care settings. Appropriate information and support should be available for those who consider but do not proceed to termination.

The Government's sexual health strategy states that no woman should wait longer than 3 weeks from the first appointment with the referring doctor to the procedure,[3] a standard supported by professional guidelines.

The RCOG's recommendations relating to the referral process include the following:

- Ideally, all women requesting termination of pregnancy are offered an assessment appointment within 5 days of referral.
- As a minimum standard, all women requesting termination of pregnancy are offered an assessment appointment within 2 weeks of referral.
- Ideally, all women can undergo the termination within 7 days of the decision to proceed being agreed.
- As a minimum standard, all women can undergo the termination within 2 weeks of the decision to proceed being agreed.
- Women should be seen as soon as possible if they require termination for urgent medical reasons.
- As a minimum standard, no woman need wait longer than 3 weeks from her initial referral to the time of termination of pregnancy.

Commissioners and providers should work together to monitor access to termination of pregnancy services and to minimise delay. All women undergoing private termination should be made aware of free access to services.

Service model

An ideal service for termination of pregnancy should provide counselling, contraceptive advice, gestational age assessment by ultrasound, a specialist nurse and a clinician for clinical assessment and management. A dedicated clinic for the support, advice and assessment of women requesting a termination is required. Clinicians caring for women requesting termination should try to identify those who require more support in decision making than can be provided in the routine clinic setting (such as those with a psychiatric history, poor social support or teenage pregnancy). Care pathways for additional support, including access to social services, should be available. Figure 6.1 shows a model care pathway.

Referrer	• GP • Family planning clinics • Young people's sexual health services • Central booking service • Genitourinary medicine or sexual health service • Self-referral • Other as designated

Information pack (referrer)	• Information for booking assessment appointment • Termination procedure options • Contacts for counselling/advice/support

Referral – assessment (see above RCOG recommendations for timescales)	• Confirm pregnancy and dates • Ultrasound • Discussion regarding options • Explain procedure • General exam for fitness • Screen for chlamydia, gonorrhoea and HIV and treat or refer to genitourinary medicine or sexual health service as appropriate • Rhesus blood group determination • Haemoglobin level determined if required • Contraception advice and discussion on long-term plans

Assessment – procedure (see above RCOG recommendations for timescales)	• Contraceptive advice and supplies provided or permanent method of contraception fitted following termination if requested by woman, including long-acting methods • Arrange post op care & follow up (if needed) • Post-termination satisfaction questionnaire

Follow up 14–21 days, subject to service-user choice	• Postoperative check • Information on counselling contacts given • Screening result given • Contraceptive advice and supplies provided or permanent method of contraception fitted following termination if requested by woman, including long-acting methods

Figure 6.1 Model care pathway for termination of pregnancy

Pre-termination care and assessment

Accurate and impartial printed information leaflets outlining the procedure and possible complications should be provided to the woman considering a termination of pregnancy before she sees the counselling doctor. Partners often accompany women to the clinic, representing an opportunity for health providers to engage them.

The assessment should include:

- a full clinical history and examination to determine fitness for the procedure
- screening, treatment and partner notification where required for *Chlamydia trachomatis* and gonorrhoeal infection
- screening for HIV and referral into appropriate sexual health clinic for treatment if results are positive
- appropriate pre-procedure blood testing: full blood count and group and save.
- a cervical smear, offered to those women who have not had one within the interval recommended in their local programme
- information about post-termination support.

Ultrasound

Accurate dating of pregnancy is an important step in assessing a woman for termination and minimising complications. All services must have access to scanning, as a part of pre-termination assessment, particularly where gestation is in doubt or where extrauterine pregnancy is suspected. All women should be scanned at the clinic visit before being seen by the doctor.

Prevention of infective complications

Care should encompass a strategy for minimising the risk of post-termination infective morbidity. Those seeking a termination of pregnancy should have their sexual health needs addressed, especially in the diagnosis and treatment of sexually transmitted infections. Screening for lower genital tract organisms, treatment and follow-up with the genitourinary clinic is ideal. As a minimum, services should offer antibiotic prophylaxis.

The RCOG recommendations relating to the regimens suitable for peri-abortion prophylaxis are:

- metronidazole 1 g rectally at the time of termination
  plus
- doxycycline 100 mg orally twice daily for 7 days, commencing on the day of termination
  or
- metronidazole 1 g rectally at the time of termination
  plus
- azithromycin 1 g orally on the day of termination.

Compliance is better with azithromycin as it is a single-dose regimen.

Obtaining valid consent

The service provider should operate a policy for obtaining consent that complies in all respects with the requirements of national minimum standards and the Private and Voluntary Healthcare (England) Regulations 2001 and any other relevant guidelines. Any competent young person, regardless of age, may independently seek medical advice and may give valid consent to medical treatment. Young women under 16 years are able to access advice and termination of pregnancy.

Informed consent for treatment must be obtained following the standard procedure of the service provider's protocol regarding consent. A consent form for the procedure should be signed at the clinic in the presence of the consulting doctor. Clinicians providing termination of pregnancy services should possess accurate knowledge about possible complications and sequelae of abortion.

Service organisation

In the absence of specific medical, social or geographical contraindications, termination of pregnancy may be managed on a daycase basis. Ideally, women admitted for termination of pregnancy should be cared for separately from other gynaecological patients. An adequate number of staffed inpatient beds must be available for those women who are unsuitable for daycase care. In a typical service, up to 5% of women will require inpatient care.

The involvement of nurses in medical abortion should be encouraged and, if future legislation permits, as recommended in the report from the House of Commons Science and Technology Committee, nurses should play a larger part in extending the availability and provision of service, including surgical procedures.[4]

Termination of pregnancy can be carried out either medically or surgically. Ideally, services should be able to offer a choice of recommended methods for each gestation band. It is essential to establish that the woman consents to the termination with a full understanding of her choices and the medical risks.

Surgical methods

Cervical priming

Cervical priming before surgical evacuation reduces the risks of cervical injury by making the cervix softer and easier to dilate. Prostaglandins remain the most widely used method of cervical preparation. Misoprostol has established a lead for cervical priming in terms of availability, ease of administration, cost and effectiveness. Cervical preparation should be routine if the woman is aged under 18 years of age or is at a gestation of more than 10 weeks.

Surgical regimens

Based on available evidence, the following regimen appears to be optimal for cervical preparation before first- or second-trimester surgical abortion. This advice is based on considerations of efficacy, adverse-effect profile and cost: misoprostol 400 micrograms (2 × 200-microgram tablets) administered vaginally, either by the woman or a clinician, 3 hours before surgery.

Conventional suction termination is an appropriate method at gestations of 7–15 weeks, although, in some settings, the skills and experience of practitioners may make medical abortion more appropriate at gestations above 12 weeks. Conventional suction termination should be avoided at gestations below 7 weeks because of the increased risk of failure and a higher incidence of failed cervical dilatation and perforation.

During suction termination, the uterus should be emptied using the suction curette and blunt forceps (if required) only. The procedure should not be completed by sharp curettage. Suction termination is usually performed under general anaesthesia. Suction termination is safer under local rather than general anaesthesia. Consideration should be given to making this option available, particularly for low-gestation procedures. For first-trimester suction termination, either electric or manual aspiration devices may be used, as both are effective and acceptable to women and clinicians. Operating times are shorter with electric aspiration.

For gestations above 15 weeks, surgical abortion by dilatation and evacuation, preceded by cervical preparation, is safe and effective when undertaken by specialist practitioners with access to the necessary instruments and who have a sufficiently large caseload to maintain their skills. A transvaginal ultrasound scan should ideally be performed after the surgical termination to confirm the completion of the procedure.

Medical methods

Medical termination of pregnancy offers a safe and acceptable non-surgical alternative to women seeking early termination of pregnancy.[5] Consideration should be given to home medical termination based on individual circumstances and choice. Medical abortion at home should be an opportunity for women applying for early pregnancy termination, as long as women are well informed and they are offered sufficient pain relief and a well-functioning follow-up programme. Medical termination can be significantly 'demedicalised': services can be offered in a nurse-led clinic and made more patient-controlled without compromising either safety or effectiveness.

Medical abortion using mifepristone plus prostaglandin is the most effective method of termination of pregnancy at gestations of less than 7 weeks.[6] Medical abortion using mifepristone plus prostaglandin continues to be an appropriate method for women in the 7–9 weeks of gestation band.

Regimens

For early medical abortion a dose of 200 mg of mifepristone, in combination with a prostaglandin, is appropriate. Based on available evidence, the following regimen appears to be optimal for early medical abortion up to 9 weeks (63 days) of gestation: mifepristone 200 mg orally followed 1–3 days later by misoprostol 800 micrograms vaginally. The misoprostol may be administered by a clinician or self-administered by the woman. For women at 49–63 days of gestation, if abortion has not occurred 4 hours after administration of misoprostol, a second dose of misoprostol 400 micrograms may be administered vaginally or orally (depending upon preference and the amount of bleeding).

For mid-trimester abortion (13–24 weeks of gestation) medical abortion with mifepristone followed by prostaglandin is an appropriate method and has been shown to be safe and effective.

An ultrasound scan should be arranged for 2 weeks after the termination, to check whether there are any retained products of conception. If products of conception are found, surgical evacuation should be arranged. Women should be advised that bleeding could be moderately heavy for 3 or 4 days, occasionally with the passage of small clots and products of conception. The bleeding may take between 1 and 3 weeks to settle completely.

Rhesus prophylaxis

Anti-D immunoglobulin G (250 iu before 20 weeks of gestation and 500 iu thereafter) should be given, by injection into the deltoid muscle, to all non-sensitised women who are RhD-negative, within 72 hours following termination of pregnancy, whether by surgical or medical methods.

Post-procedure information and follow-up

Following termination of pregnancy, women must be given a written account of the symptoms they may experience and a list of those that would make an urgent medical consultation necessary. They should be given a 24-hour telephone helpline number to use if they feel worried about pain, bleeding or high temperature. Urgent clinical assessment and emergency gynaecology admission must be available when necessary. Each woman should be offered or advised to obtain a follow-up appointment (either within the termination service or with the referring clinician) within 2 weeks of the termination. On discharge, each woman should be given a letter that includes sufficient information about the procedure to allow another practitioner elsewhere to deal with any complications.

Contraception following the procedure

Doctors should ask women if contraception was used before the unintended pregnancy. All women having termination of pregnancy should receive contraceptive advice and their choice should be clearly documented in the notes. It is essential to give information about different methods of contraception and protection against sexually transmitted diseases, as well as giving health information about using contraceptives. Immediate post-procedure counselling on contraception should be provided, to prevent a subsequent unplanned pregnancy. Quality of post-procedure care is compromised if contraception discussions are not included. Women need to be informed about how to prevent unwanted pregnancy and how soon fertility will resume. Methods should be provided at post-termination health service facilities or clients should be given a location for obtaining contraceptive supplies.

The chosen method of contraception should be initiated immediately following termination of the pregnancy. Long-acting methods should be promoted in line with NICE guidance.[7]

Pre- and post-procedure counselling

Counselling can help with the process of decision making and may assist in maintaining the woman's emotional and physical health throughout and after the procedure. Most clinicians agree that certain women need individual counselling: those who are very young, those with a history of psychiatric illness, those exhibiting extreme ambivalence and those with language or communication problems. The counsellor in the abortion clinic helps a woman to make her own decision, reinforces that decision and helps her to carry out the decision.

Special issues

Some 80% of terminations are performed in the NHS, with the majority being referred by general practitioners. Rapid access to abortion care is important to reduce the distress and complications associated with procedures undertaken at higher gestations.[8,9] Services should therefore offer arrangements that minimise delay (for example, a telephone referral system and a formal care pathway with arrangements for access from a wide range of referral sources, not just general practitioners). Appointments for assessment before termination of pregnancy can be made via a common telephone booking service which can be accessed by clients either directly or via general practitioners, family planning clinics, young people's clinics, Brook clinics and genitourinary medicine clinics. Access to termination services should be improved to include the possibility of self-referral. Fast-track referral guidelines should also be put in place for GPs and family planning services and attempts should be made to treat women undergoing termination of pregnancy separately from other gynaecological patients. Written protocols on good practice should be provided by trusts to cover all aspects of termination of pregnancy services.

Sharing of information between professionals and confidentiality

The general practitioner, referring doctor or nurse and doctor providing follow-up care should be informed in writing of the date of termination, the method used, any antibiotic treatment and medical problems, any complications or referral to other services and arrangements for contraception and follow-up. The woman's consent to passing on of information to professional carers should first be obtained, although the importance of the GP being informed in case of emergency should be emphasised to the woman. To maintain confidentiality, no information should be sent to the woman's home address unless the woman expressly wishes this.

Training needs

Training in termination of pregnancy care has become an integral part of generic and reproductive health care, with particular relevance for patient choice, communication skills and tolerance of diversity, as well as clinical and surgical care. All specialist trainees, regardless of moral or religious objections to termination of pregnancy, should fulfil the knowledge and attitude aspects of the specialist training curriculum, as indicated in the General Medical Council's guidance.[10] This guidance should be implemented and reviewed by educational leads during formative assessments. Commissioners should ensure that all aspects of the services for termination of pregnancy meet standards outlined in the RCOG guideline *The Care of Women Seeking Induced Abortion* and the RCOG's *Standards for Gynaecology*.[11]

Audit and research issues

Primary care organisations should ensure that the services provided are audited against Department of Health guidance for the registration of pregnancy advice bureaux[12] and the RCOG guideline.[2]

There are a number of issues in relation to the provision of service, such as ease of access to termination services and place of termination. Further research needs to be carried out to ascertain the optimal dosage and route of administration of misoprostol. However, pending research the recommendations set out in the RCOG guideline still stand.

References

1. Department of Health. Abortion Statistics, England and Wales 2007 [www.dh.gov.uk/en/Publicationsandstatistics/Publications/PublicationsStatistics/DH_075697].

2. Royal College of Obstetricians and Gynaecologists. *The Care of Women Requesting Induced Abortion*. National Evidence-based Clinical Guideline No. 7. London: RCOG Press; 2004.

3. Department of Health. *The National Strategy for Sexual Health and HIV*. London: DH; 2000 [www.dh.gov.uk/en/Consultations/Closedconsultations/DH_4084674].

4. House of Commons Science and Technology Committee. *Government Response to the Report from the House of Commons Science and Technology Committee on the Scientific Developments Relating to the Abortion Act 1967*. Cm 7278. London: The Stationery Office; 2007 [www.dh.gov.uk/en/Publicationsandstatistics/Publications/PublicationsPolicyAndGuidance%20/DH_080925].

5. Winikoff B. Acceptability of medical abortion in early pregnancy. *Fam Plan Perspect* 1995;27:142–8,185.

6. Peyron R, Aubény E, Targosz V, Silvestre L, Renault M, Elkik F, *et al*. Early termination of pregnancy with mifepristone (RU 486) and the orally active prostaglandin misoprostol. *N Engl J Med* 1993;328:1509–13.

7. National Collaborating Centre for Women's and Children's Health. *Long-acting Reversible Contraception: The Effective and Appropriate Use of Long-acting Reversible Contraception*. Clinical Guideline. London: RCOG Press; 2005 [guidance.nice.org.uk/CG30].

8. Buehler JW, Schulz KF, Grimes DA, Hogue CJ. The risk of serious complications from induced abortion: do personal characteristics make a difference? *Am J Obstet Gynecol* 1985;153:14–20.

9. Ferris LE, McMain-Klein M, Colodny N, Fellows GF, Lamont J. Factors associated with immediate abortion complication. *Can Med Assoc J* 1996;154:1677–85.

10. General Medical Council. *Personal Beliefs and Medical Practice*. London: GMC; 2008 [www.gmc-uk.org/guidance/ethical_guidance/personal_beliefs/Personal%20Beliefs.pdf].

11. Royal College of Obstetricians and Gynaecologists. *Standards for Gynaecology: Report of a Working Party Report*. London: RCOG Press; 2008 [www.rcog.org.uk/womens-health/clinical-guidance/standards-gynaecology].

12. Department of Health. *Procedures for the Registration of Pregnancy Advice Bureaux*. London: DH; 2001 [www.dh.gov.uk/en/Publicationsandstatistics/Publications/PublicationsPolicyAndGuidance/DH_4005566].

CHAPTER 7
Heavy menstrual bleeding

Lilantha Wedisinghe and Mary Ann Lumsden

Key points

✓ Heavy menstrual bleeding interferes with a woman's physical, social and emotional quality of life.

✓ National guidelines and standards have been produced by NICE and the RCOG. Services should be designed based on these standards to meet the public demand.

✓ There should be a dedicated, adequately equipped and staffed one-stop menstrual bleeding clinic.

✓ Although history, relevant examination, full blood count and ultrasound scan will constitute a thorough assessment, history alone is sufficient to initiate treatment in some women.

✓ The levonorgestrel-releasing intrauterine system is the first-line treatment of choice for women not wishing to conceive.

✓ Endometrial ablation or resection can be considered as a first-line treatment and the ability to perform it under local anaesthesia should be developed.

✓ A robust clinical governance framework should be in place to establish and maintain high-quality surgical, imaging, radiological and communication skills.

✓ Women should be able to access novel interventions, if appropriate. If lack of competence or resources are the issue, appropriate referral should be made.

✓ Quality control, health and safety issues and clinical risk management issues should be recognised, resolved and reported promptly.

✓ NICE has suggested several research recommendations in this important aspect of women's health.

Introduction

For clinical purposes, heavy menstrual bleeding should be defined as excessive menstrual blood loss which interferes with the woman's physical, emotional, social and sexual quality of life and which can occur alone or in combination with other symptoms. Any interventions should aim to improve quality-of-life measures.[1]

The service user's view

Women with heavy menstrual bleeding wish to have their problem taken seriously and to be part of the decision making process. They want information about all options for investigation and treatment. Many patient education websites on heavy menstrual bleeding contain an extensive analysis of available management options. The Healthcare Commission's survey programme 2004/05 on outpatient departments highlights the importance of cleanliness, discussion of the options for treatment, privacy and information on medicines. It also points out the value of informing women of 'what to expect' during and after the treatment in addition to the risks involved. Only the relevant tests should be carried out to avoid delays. Some women feel they have been forced into surgical treatment such as hysterectomy without understanding the alternatives and this is what prompted the production of the National Institute for Health and Clinical Excellence (NICE) guideline on heavy menstrual bleeding.[1]

Audits performed to examine preferences, acceptability and outcome measures of different treatments suggest that there is often a preference for them to be carried out under local anaesthesia where possible. This is particularly relevant to investigations and also the development of minimally invasive treatment options, such as endometrial ablation. However, many of these procedures are still carried out under general anaesthesia. It is also important to recognise that satisfaction rates with surgical treatment, such as hysterectomy, are extremely high.

Clinical standards and national guidelines

Standards for Gynaecology,[2] published by the RCOG in 2008, defined expected national clinical standards. Standards for patient safety, the top priority in clinical care, is considered as a national standard in risk management for maternity and gynaecology.[3]

The NICE guideline on heavy menstrual bleeding provides the most up-to-date evidence-based recommendations both on provision of care and the areas that need to be researched further. The content of this chapter is based largely on the NICE guideline.[1] NICE also produces guidance relating to interventional procedures, as well as technology appraisals relating to specific techniques. Examples of relevant techniques are endometrial ablation, including fluid-filled thermal balloon, microwave, free fluid thermal, impedance control and endometrial cryotherapy, uterine artery embolisation, laparoscopic laser myomectomy, hysteroscopic laser myomectomy and laparoscopic hysterectomy. Recommendations of the NICE guidelines on long-acting reversible contraception,[4] osteoporosis[5] and the referral guidelines for suspected cancer[6] also provide relevant information concerning specific areas that maybe of relevance.

Service model and care pathways

Before her outpatient appointment, the woman should receive information that will form the basis for discussion and informed choice. This should cover the indication, procedure description, recovery time, post-procedural effects and the balance of risks and benefits. Clinicians should work in partnership with women to support informed choice. Whether heavy menstrual blood loss is a problem should be determined not by measuring blood loss but by the women herself.[1] Final treatment decision should be based on the care pathway (Figure 7.1) and consideration of the potential risks and benefits (Table 7.1).

Taking a history is vital for the diagnosis and management of heavy menstrual bleeding. If the history indicates uncomplicated heavy menstrual bleeding and where structural or histological abnormality is unlikely to be present, pharmaceutical treatment can be started straightaway. Otherwise, examination and investigations should be performed. A physical examination should be carried out before investigating for structural or histological abnormalities and fitting a levonorgestrel-releasing intrauterine system (LNG-IUS). Ultrasound scan should be carried out if:

- there is an abnormal bleeding pattern
- the body build precludes sufficient bimanual examination
- the uterus is palpable abdominally
- a pelvic mass of uncertain origin is detected
- the medical treatment fails.

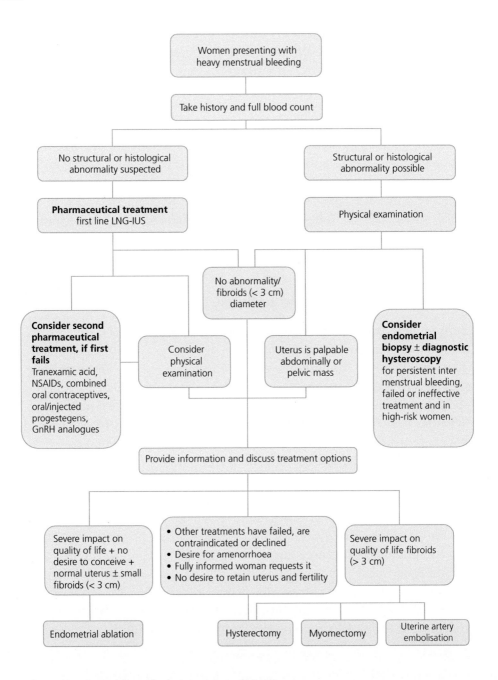

Figure 7.1 Care pathway for heavy menstrual bleeding

Table 7.1 Potential risks and benefits of treatments for heavy menstrual bleeding (adapted from NICE guideline on heavy menstrual bleeding)[1]

Intervention	Benefits		Potential unwanted outcomes experienced by some women[a]
LNG-IUS	Fertility is reversed after removal; therapeutic effect on endometriosis; minimal systemic adverse effects; does not interact with liver enzyme inducing agents; lasts 3 years; cost effective	C	Irregular bleeding that may last for over 6 months; hormone-related problems such as breast tenderness, acne or headaches, which, if present, are generally minor and transient
		LC	Amenorrhoea
		R	Uterine perforation at the time of LNG-IUS insertion
Tranexamic acid	Does not interfere with fertility; only needs to be taken during heavy menstrual bleeding; acts within 3 hours of administration; where hormonal treatments are not acceptable	LC	Indigestion; diarrhoea; headaches
NSAIDs	Do not interfere with fertility; only need to be taken for 3–5 days; useful where hormonal treatments are not acceptable to the woman; inexpensive	C	Indigestion; diarrhoea
		R	Worsening of asthma in sensitive individuals; peptic ulcers with possible bleeding and peritonitis
Combined oral contraceptives	Very effective and acceptable contraceptive	C	Mood changes; headaches; nausea; fluid retention; breast tenderness
		R	Deep vein thrombosis; stroke; heart attack
Oral progestogen	Can be used where estrogen treatment is contraindicated	C	Weight gain; bloating; breast tenderness; headaches; acne (all are minor and transient)
		R	Depression
Injected progestogen	Can be used where estrogen treatment is contraindicated; long lasting; therapeutic effect on endometriosis	C	Weight gain; irregular bleeding; amenorrhoea; premenstrual-like syndrome
		LC	Small loss of bone mineral density: largely recovered when treatment is discontinued
GnRHa	Effectively reduces pain associated with endometriosis	C	Menopausal-like symptoms (such as hot flushes, increased sweating, vaginal dryness)
		LC	Osteoporosis, particularly trabecular bone with longer than 6 months of use

Table 7.1 (continued)

Intervention	Benefits	Potential unwanted outcomes experienced by some women[a]	
Endometrial ablation	Less invasive than radical surgery; can be performed without general or regional anaesthesia; possible elimination of bleeding	C	Vaginal discharge; increased period pain or cramping (even if no further bleeding); need for additional surgery
		LC	Infection
		R	Perforation (but very rare with second-generation techniques)
Uterine artery embolisation	Potentially sparing effect of fertility; can be performed under local anaesthesia; rapid response	C	Persistent vaginal discharge; post-embolisation syndrome (pain, nausea, vomiting and fever) not involving hospitalisation)
		LC	Need for additional surgery; premature ovarian failure, particularly in a woman over 45 years of age; haematoma
		R	Haemorrhage; non-target embolisation causing tissue necrosis; infection causing septicaemia
Myomectomy	Potentially sparing effect of fertility; reduces symptoms associated with fibroids	LC	Adhesions (which may lead to pain and/or impaired fertility); need for additional surgery; recurrence of fibroids; perforation (hysteroscopic route); infection
		R	Haemorrhage
Hysterectomy	Complete elimination of menstrual bleeding and uterine pathology	C	Infection
		LC	Intraoperative haemorrhage; damage to other abdominal organs, such as the urinary tract or bowel; urinary dysfunction: frequent passing of urine and incontinence
		R	Venous thromboembolism (deep vein thrombosis and pulmonary embolism)
		VR	Death
Oophorectomy at the time of hysterectomy	Complete elimination of ovarian pathology; elimination of symptoms associated with premenstrual syndrome	C	Menopausal symptoms

[a] Common (C) = 1/100 chance, less common (LC) = 1/1000 chance, rare (R) = 1/10,000 chance, very rare (VR) = 1/100,000 chance

Persistent intermenstrual bleeding, failed or ineffective treatment or the presence of other risk factors are indications for an endometrial biopsy to exclude endometrial atypical hyperplasia or carcinoma.[2] Diagnostic hysteroscopy should be considered if the suspicion of endometrial cancer is high; for example, in the presence of risk factors such as polycystic ovary syndrome or obesity or if a woman is taking tamoxifen.

Pharmaceutical treatment

Pharmaceutical treatment is the treatment of choice for many women with heavy menstrual bleeding and the type often depends on whether she desires fertility. Pharmaceutical treatment should be considered where no structural or histological abnormality is present or any fibroids are less than 3 cm in diameter and do not distort the uterine cavity. The acceptability of hormonal contraception to women with heavy menstrual bleeding should be discussed.

If the history or investigations indicate that any pharmaceutical treatment is acceptable, treatment options should be considered in the following order:[1]

1. LNG-IUS
2. tranexamic acid or nonsteroidal anti-inflammatory drugs (NSAIDs) or combined oral contraceptives
3. norethisterone 5 mg three times a day from day 5 to day 26 of the menstrual cycle or injected long-acting progestogens.

If hormonal treatments are not acceptable, then either tranexamic acid and/or NSAIDs can be used. The same regimen can be used while definitive treatment is awaited. Continued use of tranexamic acid and/or NSAIDs is recommended for as long as they are found to be beneficial by the woman. However, they should be discontinued if they do not improve symptoms within three menstrual cycles.

The LNG-IUS often results in changes in bleeding pattern in the first few cycles, which may last more than 6 months. Women should be advised accordingly.

In women who have uterine fibroids and heavy menstrual bleeding, gonadotrophin-releasing hormone analogue (GnRHa) could be considered before surgery or when all other treatment options for uterine fibroids are contraindicated. Add-back therapy is recommended to counteract adverse effects or if the GnRHa is to be used more than 6 months.

Endometrial ablation should be considered in women who do not want to conceive in the future. However, they must be advised to avoid subsequent pregnancy and on the need of effective contraception, if required. All women suitable for endometrial ablation should have access to a second-generation ablation technique. However, first-generation ablation techniques, such as rollerball endometrial ablation and transcervical resection of the endometrium, are appropriate if hysteroscopic myomectomy is to be carried out at the same time.[1]

Uterine artery embolisation is effective in decreasing menstrual blood loss and is indicated for women with heavy menstrual bleeding associated with uterine fibroids and who want to retain their uterus and/or to avoid surgery.[7] Women should be adequately counselled about possible post-procedure complications so that potentially serious complications, such as infection, can be recognised. The lack of information regarding the impact on future fertility should also be emphasised if relevant.

Hysterectomy should not be offered as a first-line treatment solely for heavy menstrual bleeding. However, hysterectomy should be considered when other treatments have failed, are contraindicated or are declined by properly counselled women. Counselling should include: the impact on fertility, sexual feelings and bladder function; treatment complications; the need for further treatment; alternative surgery; the psychosocial impact of hysterectomy; the woman's expectations. The route of choice for hysterectomy is vaginal, with abdominal hysterectomy as a second choice. Laparoscopy-assisted vaginal hysterectomy should be considered when there is a need for oophorectomy during vaginal hysterectomy or where there are technical issues, such as morbid obesity and adhesions, when referral to an appropriately trained specialist maybe required. Individual assessment is necessary when deciding the route for hysterectomy. The assessment should include uterine size, the presence and size of fibroids, mobility and descent of the uterus, size and shape of the vagina, outcomes of previous surgery and the presence of other gynaecological condition or disease.[1]

Healthy ovaries should not routinely be removed at the time of hysterectomy for heavy menstrual bleeding.

There should be up-to-date local guidelines and robust mechanisms to prevent infection and venous thromboembolism for women undergoing major surgical treatment for heavy menstrual bleeding.

Staff and training implications

All health professionals undertaking surgical or radiological procedures to diagnose and treat heavy menstrual bleeding should demonstrate their technical and counselling competence, either during their training or during subsequent practice.[1] There should be robust clinical governance frameworks to maintain high-quality surgical, imaging and radiological skills. A structured process of formal assessment can be used for this purpose through recognised training schemes.

With rapid advances in gynaecological surgical technology, working hour restrictions, women with increasingly complex problems and concerns about the quality of care, new methods of surgical education must be adopted to ensure the competency of trainees.[8] Research suggests that laboratory-based surgical training allows trainees to learn in a low-stress environment where mistakes are permissible, procedures can be repeated multiple times to improve muscle memory and formative feedback can more rapidly lead to competence. With ever-increasing demand for minimal access surgery, including interventions for heavy menstrual bleeding, laboratory-based surgical training should be promoted and the availability for such training courses maximised.

Strategies for improving the clinical learning environment,[9] such as inter-professional learning and 'taster sessions' are available and authorities must be encouraged to establish them where possible, to exceed a minimum set of criteria.

Opportunities for specialist training

The operative competence of healthcare professionals who acquire new skills in procedures relating to heavy menstrual bleeding should be formally assessed by their trainers through a structured process. These have been defined within training schemes of RCOG, the Royal College of Radiologists and the Society and College of Radiographers.

Specialty trainees should be supported by providing access to the Advanced Training Skills Modules on benign abdominal surgery, benign vaginal surgery, benign gynaecological surgery: laparoscopy and benign gynaecological surgery: hysteroscopy.

Laboratory-based surgical training could be useful, not only for trainees but also for specialists, to identify more effective methods and to develop better techniques that will be beneficial for the patients for whom they care.

The LNG-IUS is the first line of treatment for heavy menstrual bleeding. Owing to its efficiency as a contraceptive, its availability within primary care setting should save costs, time and the resources of both the woman and the service provider. It will also improve acceptability, since there should be at least one general practitioner in every practice who has the skills to fit the device. It is, therefore, important to review local provision and the special skills needed for effective use of the LNG-IUS. Consequently, particular emphasis should be made regarding general practice training. Only a small proportion of GP trainees get clinical experience in obstetrics and gynaecology and it is probable that these people will be best placed to become certified to insert the LNG-IUS. The Faculty of Sexual and Reproductive Healthcare provides appropriate training and maintains its diplomates' competencies in a structured programme.

Resource implications

There should be a dedicated one-stop clinic for those with heavy menstrual bleeding, with facilities within the clinic for diagnostic and therapeutic gynaecology, including hysteroscopy and pelvic ultrasound scanning.[2,10] Adequately trained health professionals should be available for counselling, assessment, insertion of the LNG-IUS and, possibly, provision of techniques such as endometrial ablation. The role of a gynaecological nurse specialist in facilitating initial assessment and post-treatment follow-up, which includes the provision of telephone advice, can be very useful for women with heavy menstrual bleeding. Care pathways should be designed to ensure ready access for those who have an abnormal histological diagnosis.

Novel minimal access surgical methods can be very expensive. They attract the public mostly because of the 'user-friendly' nature of such methods: less pain, quick recovery and, hence, shorter hospital stay. However, long-term cost effectiveness is less certain and appropriately skilled individuals must be available for the treatment of fibroid-associated heavy menstrual bleeding.

Uterine artery embolisation is becoming an increasingly popular intervention. It minimises heavy menstrual bleeding quickly and may be the only option for women who are not fit for general or regional anaesthesia. It is ideal to make this option available, together with second-generation ablation techniques, in every gynaecological centre that offers services for heavy menstrual bleeding. Referral pathways should be agreed locally and reviewed annually.

Advanced training should ensure competency in complex procedures and should be located in centres with sufficient workload to allow adequate experience of these procedures.

Audit and other clinical governance issues

New therapeutic products and techniques for investigation should be made available for patients and the local clinical governance framework must ensure this. It should also make sure that service providers are trained to offer new services competently, effectively and safely.

Clinical governance policies should be able to monitor treatment complications, patient choice, patient satisfaction and uptake rate. A critical incident reporting system should ensure that all relevant incidents are reported promptly, locally and nationally, as appropriate. Staff involvement in risk management exercises should be monitored to ensure that appropriate incident forms have been completed and that the staff involved have received feedback.

Staff knowledge and compliance with up-to-date clinical guidelines can be audited as well as activities such as the taking of consent, especially for complex procedures.

Quality control and health and safety issues relating to novel products should be appropriately dealt with. Adverse outcomes of unexpected adverse events, endometrial ablation and other treatments should be reported locally and to the National Patient Safety Agency, Medicines and Healthcare products Regulatory Agency, the unexpected adverse events registry and other relevant authorities.[3]

Established healthcare professionals should be able to demonstrate that their current practice and competency meet or exceed the standard of newly trained professionals. If a particular healthcare professional lacks the competence to undertake a procedure, referral to a skilled professional should be made. Similarly, if an organisation is under-resourced, then referral to a well-resourced centre should be made. The lead clinicians and organisations that commission services should be responsible for recognising and negotiating such requirements.

Radiologists should be able to demonstrate their consultation and technical competence. Outcomes of radiological interventions should be audited and should be available to gynaecologists, who usually initiate the therapeutic decision.

If there are concerns about an individual doctor's performance or the gynaecology service as a whole, the services of an RCOG external clinical advisory team can be sought. The guidance provides relevant advice for such a referral, which includes the role of the General Medical Council, National Clinical Assessment Service and the Healthcare Commission.[11]

Research recommendations

NICE has recognised important areas that need further research and development.

Risk factors for heavy menstrual bleeding and uterine pathology

Epidemiology of women presenting with heavy menstrual bleeding in primary care.

Impact of heavy menstrual bleeding on quality of life.

The currently available heavy menstrual bleeding-specific health-related quality-of-life measures need to be validated.

Heavy menstrual bleeding-specific quality-of-life measures need to be developed for use in research and clinical practice.

Need for more research on the interaction of ethnicity and the perception of heavy menstrual bleeding.

Measurement of menstrual blood loss

Investigation of routine use of indirect measurements of menstrual blood loss in primary and secondary care.

Need for quality-of-life research in heavy menstrual bleeding and menstruation.

Investigations for structural and histological abnormalities

The production of predictive values for heavy menstrual bleeding and significant uterine pathology in primary care populations.

Pharmaceutical treatments

A study to investigate the use of LNG-IUS in fibroids larger than 3 cm.

A study to examine the association between size and site of uterine fibroids and heavy menstrual bleeding.

Non-hysterectomy surgery for heavy menstrual bleeding

Endometrial ablation

Where evidence is not available on endometrial thinning prior to different ablative techniques, it is recommended that this research be undertaken.

A randomised controlled trial of the clinical effectiveness and cost effectiveness of the various second-generation ablation techniques against one another.

An opportunity to evaluate any new endometrial ablation techniques within a randomised controlled trial format.

Further interventions for uterine fibroids associated with heavy menstrual bleeding

The effect of uterine artery embolisation and myomectomy on the long-term fertility of women.

The psychosexual impacts of uterine artery embolisation and myomectomy.

The long-term recurrence rates of fibroids after uterine artery embolisation or myomectomy.

How uterine artery embolisation affects blood flow in the uterus.

The mechanism of action by which uterine artery embolisation reduces menstrual blood loss.

Ovarian function after uterine artery embolisation or myomectomy.

The ovarian and uterine function of women with or without heavy menstrual bleeding.

Hysterectomy

An investigation into the medium- and long-term outcomes of subtotal and total hysterectomy.

An investigation into the effect of hysterectomy and oophorectomy on cancer.

Competencies

The existence of volume–outcome relationships in gynaecological procedures, taking into account case mix, hospital and surgeon factors.

Reference

1. National Collaborating Centre for Women's and Children's Health. *Heavy Menstrual Bleeding*. London: RCOG Press; 2007 [http://guidance.nice.org.uk/CG44].
2. Royal College of Obstetricians and Gynaecologists. *Standards for Gynaecology: Report of a Working Party*. London: RCOG Press; 2008 [www.rcog.org.uk/womens-health/clinical-guidance/standards-gynaecology].
3. Royal College of Obstetricians and Gynaecologists. *Improving Patient Safety: Risk Management for Maternity and Gynaecology*. Clinical Governance Advice No. 2. London: RCOG; 2005 [www.rcog.org.uk/womens-health/clinical-guidance/improving-patient-safety-risk-management-maternity-and-gynaecology].
4. National Collaborating Centre for Women's and Children's Health. *Long-acting Reversible Contraception: The Effective and Appropriate Use of Long-acting Reversible Contraception*. Clinical Guideline. London: RCOG Press; 2005 [guidance.nice.org.uk/CG30].
5. National Institute for Health and Clinical Excellence. Osteoporosis: assessment of fracture risk and the prevention of osteoporotic fractures in individuals at high risk. [http://guidance.nice.org.uk/CG/Wave7/32].
6. National Collaborating Centre for Primary Care. *Referral Guidelines for Suspected Cancer in Adults and Children*. London: Royal College of General Practitioners; 2005 [http://guidance.nice.org.uk/CG27/Guidance/pdf/English].
7. Royal College of Radiologists, Royal College of Obstetricians and Gynaecologists. Clinical *Recommendations on the Use of Uterine Artery Embolisation in the Management of Fibroids: Report of a Joint Working Party*. London: RCOG Press; 2000.
8. Goff BA. Changing the paradigm in surgical education. *Obstet Gynecol* 2008;112:328–32.
9. Royal College of Obstetricians and Gynaecologists, Royal College of Midwives. *The Clinical Learning Environment and Recruitment: Report of a Joint Working Party*. London: RCOG Press; 2008 [www.rcog.org.uk/womens-health/clinical-guidance/clinical-learning-environment-and-recruitment-report-joint-working-p].
10. Abu JI, Habiba MA, Baker R, Halligan AW, Naftalin NJ, Hsu R, *et al*. Quantitative and qualitative assessment of women's experience of a one-stop menstrual clinic in comparison with traditional gynaecology clinics. *BJOG* 2001;108:993–9.
11. Royal College of Obstetricians and Gynaecologists. *Performance and Service Reviews Part 1: Policy: Report of an RCOG Working Party*. London: RCOG Press; 2007 [www.rcog.org.uk/womens-health/clinical-guidance/performance-and-service-reviews-part-1-policy].

CHAPTER 8
Post-reproductive gynaecology

Ailsa Gebbie and Margaret Rees

Key points

- ✓ Post-reproductive care needs to be coordinated by a regional specialist team integrating primary and secondary care.
- ✓ Care should not be delivered in general gynaecological clinics by mainstream gynaecologists.
- ✓ Specialist care can be delivered in a variety of settings: hospital, community-based sexual and reproductive healthcare clinics and outreach services in primary care.
- ✓ A local lead clinician should be identified, who may be a hospital gynaecologist, sexual and reproductive health specialist or general practitioner with a special interest.
- ✓ Medical and nursing staff need to be trained and to maintain expertise through regular attendance at updating courses.
- ✓ Job plans need to include time for continuing training and for liaison between primary and secondary care.
- ✓ Dedicated telephone, answerphone and email contact systems for women and health professionals need to be maintained.
- ✓ The specialist team needs to link with allied health professionals who are involved in the care of postmenopausal women, such as radiographers, physiotherapists and continence advisors.
- ✓ The specialist team need to link with other specialties such as endocrinology, oncology, fertility and rheumatology to provide a 'one stop' service for women with special needs, such as early menopause, estrogen-dependent cancer and osteoporosis.
- ✓ A regional database of women with a premature menopause should be in place and these women should normally be offered HRT until the average age of the menopause (51 years).

▓ Introduction

The menopause can now be considered to be a mid-life event as the lifespan of women in the UK continues to increase. Many women now survive well into their tenth decade. Thus, both the short- and long-term problems of the menopause, both for the women themselves and for society, are key issues for health professionals. The multifaceted 'model of care' concept defining how health services are delivered for the menopausal woman is a model integrating primary and secondary care to deal with the multiple problems which can affect post-reproductive health.

In the UK, unless surgery is required, most post-reproductive gynaecological care is delivered in the primary care setting. Only women with complex issues or who fail to respond to treatment are referred to specialist services. Currently, there are few NHS dedicated clinics for post-reproductive health. These are located either in hospitals or, increasingly, in community-based sexual and reproductive health services; consequently, general gynaecologists may be delivering this service, with resulting concerns about expertise and training. The RCOG *Standards for Gynaecology* specifies that post-reproductive health should be managed by a dedicated team.[1]

▓ The service user's view

Based on telephone and internet surveys, it is apparent that women want clear, evidence-based information about the various hormonal and non-hormonal treatment options.[2,3] They feel that media reports have generally exaggerated the risks of hormone replacement therapy (HRT) and that not enough information is available about alternative and complementary therapies. Although the most common reason for seeking medical help is for relief of menopausal symptoms, one internet survey showed that only 20% of sufferers had discussed their symptoms with health professionals and only 12% were using prescribed treatment.[3] It is well known that women do not seek help for symptoms of urogenital atrophy and will suffer distressing symptoms in silence, often through embarrassment.

It can be difficult for women to find balanced information on the menopause and HRT. Several UK clinician-led websites have been developed and can be easily accessed on the internet.[4] Similarly, accurate and unbiased information leaflets are often not easily found. The UK

Medicines and Healthcare products Regulatory Authority (MHRA) has produced patient information leaflets in response to HRT publicity, which healthcare professionals can print off and give to women.[5]

Clinical standards and national guidelines

Clinical standards and guidelines are available from the RCOG, the MHRA, the British Menopause Society, the National Osteoporosis Guideline Group and Clinical Knowledge Summaries.[1,5,6,7,8] These detail standards for primary care and dedicated specialist services, dealing with premature menopause and management of women at high risk of osteoporotic fracture.

Current standards and guidelines clearly outline therapeutic strategies, with their benefits and risks, as well as the role of alternative and complementary therapies. The overall evidence from randomised trials of the effect of alternative and complementary therapies on menopausal symptoms is largely that of a placebo benefit.

Women with premature menopause are advised to take HRT until their early 50s, which is the average age of the normal menopause. Findings from trials and studies in older women should not be extrapolated to them. The MHRA issued clear guidance that HRT was not a first-line agent for the treatment or prevention of osteoporosis in women after the age of normal menopause, as the overall risks outweighed the benefits.[5]

Service model and care pathways

The UK model of care for post-reproductive gynaecology is that most women will seek advice in the primary care setting. Only women with complex problems need referral to a specialist hospital or community-based sexual and reproductive healthcare service. Well-developed specialist services will support primary care colleagues with regular updating meetings, telephone and email advice and providing patient information leaflets.

Care pathways are available from the organisations detailed above. A suggested care pathway is detailed below for healthy postmenopausal women and is suitable for primary care (Figure 8.1). Women with specialist needs or abnormal bleeding need referral to a dedicated service and indications for referral are listed in Table 8.1.

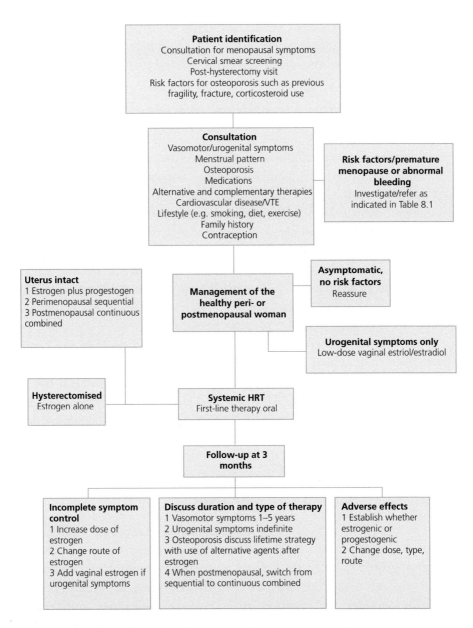

Figure 8.1 Care pathway for the management of menopause

The model of service may include patient support groups, with nurses and clinicians acting as facilitators. These groups can be targeted either at all menopausal women or at specific groups, such as those with

Table 8.1 Indications for post-reproductive referral and the information that needs to made available to the specialist service

Indication	Definition/symptoms	Information/investigation to be included in referral letter, if available
Abnormal bleeding	Non-HRT users: e.g. a sudden change in menstrual pattern, intermenstrual bleeding, postcoital bleeding or a postmenopausal bleed	Ultrasound scan, ideally transvaginal, reporting endometrial thickness Cervical smear result and date Examination findings
	HRT users: Sequential HRT: change in pattern of withdrawal bleeds or breakthrough bleeding	
	Continuous combined or long-cycle regimens: breakthrough bleeding persisting for more than 4–6 months after starting or which is not lessening; a bleed after amenorrhoea on a continuous combined regimen	
Multiple treatment failure	3 or more regimens tried	List types of HRT and detail problems
Cardiovascular disease	Venous thromboembolism (confirmed), family history of unprovoked event in a first-degree relative age less than 50 years	Confirmation of history, e.g. venogram, ultrasound, V/Q scan, anticoagulation history, circumstance of event, thrombophilia screen
	Ischaemic heart disease or stroke	Confirmation of history, drug history, blood pressure, relevant family history
Premature menopause	Menopause at under 40 years of age	Reason for ovarian failure; follicle-stimulating hormone, thyroid function test, bone mineral density, autoantibody screen
Osteoporosis (treatment and prevention)	Confirmed or high risk, e.g. early menopause, corticosteroids > 5 mg prednisolone/day, positive family history, especially first-degree relative, low body mass index	Bone mineral density by DXA with T & Z scores History of traumatic/non-traumatic fracture
Previous or high risk of hormone-dependent malignancy	e.g. breast ± ovarian, endometrial cancer	Details of disease: stage, treatment, family history

premature menopause. Patient support groups can be either in primary or secondary care.

Staff and training implications

Care needs to be provided by a multidisciplinary team involving:

- a lead clinician (gynaecologist, sexual and reproductive health specialist or GP with a special interest) who holds appropriate national qualification or other recognised certificate, with support from other appropriately qualified clinicians to cover for training, leave and other absences
- a specialist nurse(s) who can run independent clinics supported by the clinicians.

The clinicians and nurse(s) need to maintain dedicated telephone, answerphone and email contact systems for women and health professionals. Staff need to liaise with other allied health professionals who are involved in the care of postmenopausal women, such as radiographers, physiotherapists and continence advisors. Other specialties, such as endocrinology, oncology, fertility and rheumatology, need to be linked into the service to provide a 'one stop' service for women with special needs, such as early menopause, estrogen-dependent cancer and osteoporosis. Continuing training will need to be coordinated by the lead clinician to ensure that staff are providing evidence-based advice. This may comprise regular staff meetings with case discussions and opportunities to attend national updating conferences.

Opportunities for specialist training

Specialist training for doctors is available through an RCOG Advanced Training Skills Module and a Special Skills Module of the Faculty of Sexual and Reproductive Health. These have been developed in conjunction with guidance from the British Menopause Society. Menopause care will be an integral component of the new specialty training for the sexual and reproductive health curriculum which is currently under development. Specialist training for nurses is through the Royal College of Nursing and various distance learning opportunities, such as the Oxford Menopause Course. Expertise for all healthcare professionals needs to maintained by regular attendance at training and updating courses.

Resource implications

Each health authority or region should have a dedicated menopause clinic, so the major resource implication is in funding and supporting a specific clinical team outside the routine gynaecological service. Patient flow needs to be regularly mapped so that bottlenecks can be identified and dealt with within established referral timescales. This may lead to a different model of delivering specialist care, such as an outreach clinic in primary care rather than in hospital. Time needs to be made available in job plans so that members of the specialist team can undertake teaching in primary care on a regular basis.

Audit and research

A variety of projects can be undertaken:

- number of new referrals to each clinic, together with the reasons for referral
- database of number of women with premature ovarian failure on HRT and their long-term outcome data (including osteoporosis, cardiovascular disease and fertility)
- uptake rates of different treatments and complications reported (type of hormonal, medical and alternative treatments)
- appropriate use of investigations (such as endocrine investigations, bone density scans and endometrial biopsies)
- patient satisfaction surveys.

References

1. Royal College of Obstetricians and Gynaecologists. *Standards for Gynaecology. Report of a Working Party*. London: RCOG Press; 2008 [www.rcog.org.uk/womens-health/clinical-guidance/standards-gynaecology].
2. Williams RE, Kalilani L, DiBenedetti DB, Zhou X, Fehnel SE, Clark RV. Healthcare seeking and treatment for menopausal symptoms in the United States. *Maturitas* 2007;58:348–58.
3. Cumming GP, Herald J, Moncur R, Currie H, Lee AJ. Women's attitudes to hormone replacement therapy, alternative therapy and sexual health: a web-based survey. *Menopause Int* 2007;13:79–83.
4. Menopause Matters: an independent clinician-led website [www.menopausematters.co.uk].
5. Medicines and Healthcare products Regulatory Agency. Hormone-replacement therapy [www.mhra.gov.uk/Safetyinformation/Generalsafetyinformationandadvice/

Product-specificinformationandadvice/Hormonereplacementtherapy(HRT)/
CON019593].

6. British Menopause Society [www.thebms.org.uk].

7. National Osteoporosis Guideline Group [www.shef.ac.uk/NOGG].

8. NHS Clinical Knowledge Summaries. Menopause management [http://cks.library.nhs.uk/menopause].

CHAPTER 9

Urogynaecology

Robert Freeman and Ash Monga

Key points

✓ The RCOG standards for urogynaecology provide a basic set of essentials that are necessary to provide our patients with a consistently high quality of care, irrespective of where that care is provided. Implementation with the support of national guidelines, audit and clinical governance should help to achieve this aim.

✓ Clinicians, with trust support, should engage with continence advisory services, general practitioners and primary care trusts to ensure that initial management of incontinence and pelvic organ prolapse is undertaken in primary care, in line with National Institute for Health and Clinical Excellence guidelines, and that locally agreed referral pathways are in place.

✓ There should be comprehensive written information about pelvic floor dysfunction to help women to make informed choices about management options.

✓ Clinicians should establish dedicated urogynaecology clinics and multidisciplinary teams in secondary care, with regular multidisciplinary team meetings.

✓ In selected centres, such as tertiary referral centres, more extensive multidisciplinary team meetings, with urological and coloproctology input, should be established, with appropriate investigatory and surgical skills available.

✓ Appropriate training, either subspecialty or ATSM, and sufficient workload to maintain surgical competence should be available (the methods of surgical assessment need further evaluation).

✓ All women undergoing prolapse or incontinence surgery should be included in national audit strategies, such as the British Society of Urogynaecology's surgical audit database, following informed consent.

✓ Clinicians should inform clinical governance leads when undertaking new surgical procedures.

Introduction

Urinary incontinence, prolapse and anal incontinence have, not surprisingly, a significant impact on quality of life, affecting relationships, social and physical activities, work and body image and thus resulting in psychological distress and the development of coping strategies. Significant advances have been made in the understanding of these symptoms and conditions, their investigation and treatment. The RCOG's clinical standards for urogynaecology have been jointly developed with the British Society of Urogynaecology (BSUG) to provide a framework that should ensure best and evidence-based practice. It is important that these standards are appropriately adopted by clinicians to improve the quality of care for our patients.

The service user's view

The wishes of patients have been paramount in the development of the NHS 18-week referral-to-treatment interval and these should allow quick access to specialist services where indicated.[1] However, as discussed below, the initial management of pelvic floor dysfunction should take place in primary care[2] and locally agreed referral pathways are recommended.

Within both primary and secondary care there should be good verbal and written information about pelvic floor dysfunction to enable women to make informed choices about their care and management options: conservative, surgical and medical. These should include success rates, operation-specific complications and the adverse effects of drug therapy. Women should also have the opportunity for follow-up consultations with a specialist if required.

For treatments, it is important that both women and clinicians have realistic expectations of outcome. Interestingly, it has been shown that not all women expect a complete cure, with the majority, in one study of women with urinary incontinence, 'wanting a good improvement so that the symptoms no longer interfere with their life'.[3]

When assessing outcomes, studies suggest that patient satisfaction and objective measures are regarded as the most important by clinicians,[4] while for women, 'symptom relief' is the most commonly cited treatment 'goal' with 'physical appearance' being the least important.[5] For the latter, (in relation to prolapse surgery), in an editorial in the *New England*

Journal of Medicine, Rogers quoted: 'few women care what their vaginas look like; more are concerned with restoring bowel, bladder and sexual functions'.[6] It might be more important therefore to regard the patient's opinion of functionality as the main measure of outcome rather than the anatomical result of surgery. To determine whether success has been achieved, preoperative expectations and goals should be recorded and reviewed on follow-up. The acronym of 'EGGS' has been proposed as a method of achieving this: Expectations, Goal setting, Goal achievement and Satisfaction.[7] This measure has been shown to be useful in clinical practice.[8]

It is becoming evident that many women want to know the efficacy and safety of treatments, with particular emphasis on surgery. Audit data are therefore important when counselling patients, who should have information on their clinician's outcomes as well as national data. These data can be collected via the BSUG surgical audit database for urinary incontinence and prolapse.[9]

Clinical standards and national guidelines

The National Institute for Health and Clinical Excellence (NICE) has produced the most comprehensive, up-to-date guidelines for the management of urinary incontinence and these are strongly recommended for clinical practice.[2] Implementation advice is also provided, including continuity of care and multi-agency issues, resources, training and competence. In Scotland, the Scottish Intercollegiate Guidelines Network (SIGN) provide similar recommendations.[10] NICE also makes several recommendations on the use of mesh in prolapse surgery. [11] Before introducing these techniques to their practice, clinicians should:

- inform clinical governance leads
- ensure that patients understand the uncertainty of the long-term results and complications
- provide patients with clear written information
- audit and review clinical outcomes of all patients having mesh procedures for prolapse.

Arguably, these recommendations are applicable to the introduction of all new surgical procedures but for use of vaginal mesh for prolapse surgery, especially for primary cases, caution is recommended until audit data and the results of clinical trials are available. As the review commissioned by NICE commented, 'the evidence for most efficacy and safety outcomes was too sparse to provide meaningful conclusions about the use of mesh/graft in anterior and/or posterior vaginal wall prolapse surgery'.[12]

In addition to these guidelines, valuable information is available from the International Continence Society[13] and the International Urogynecological Association[14] on standardisation of terminology.

Standards for initial management

The initial assessment and management of women with urinary incontinence is detailed in the NICE and SIGN guidelines and these are equally applicable to all pelvic floor disorders, including prolapse, anal and faecal incontinence, with a specific NICE guideline being available for the latter.[15] Streamlining assessment and management is vital and much of this can take place in the primary care setting. As mentioned, locally agreed referral pathways should be in place after discussion with general practitioners, continence advisory services and primary care trusts.

A careful history should be taken, including the use of symptom and quality-of-life questionnaires to assess severity and worry for the woman (such as the International Consultation on Incontinence questionnaires).[16]

Explanations, both written, verbal and website information should be given. Detailed recommendations for examination and investigations are provided by NICE[2] and SIGN[10] and it is important to emphasise that pathology should be excluded, such as a pelvic mass, neuropathy or bladder tumour (by investigation of microscopic haematuria).

Following investigation, NICE recommends, as initial therapy for urinary incontinence, pelvic floor muscle training for a minimum of 3 months and other conservative measures such as lifestyle management and bladder retraining. These steps should be undertaken in primary care through community continence services, although if these are unavailable, they may be carried out in the secondary care setting. If this initial conservative treatment is unsuccessful, referral back to the GP is indicated for possible drug treatment for overactive bladder symptoms or to a specialist in secondary care for possible persistent stress urinary incontinence and/or pelvic organ prolapse. All of these services should be evidence-based and of the same recommended standard, whoever provides the service.

Model service and care pathways

Referral pathways and protocols for local use can be adapted from those recommended by NICE and one example of this adaptation is shown in Figure 9.1.

In secondary care, clinicians should either undertake a dedicated clinic. Alternatively, a significant proportion of their work should involve women with urogynaecological problems. The numbers referred and seen should be audited annually to assess caseload.

There should be facilities for the full range of investigations, including urodynamics, anorectal physiology and imaging, where appropriate. There should be multidisciplinary clinics with urology colleagues for complex incontinence problems and with coloproctologists for women with concomitant anal incontinence, as well as the opportunity to follow-up those with obstetric anal sphincter injuries. In addition, collaboration with continence advisors, physiotherapists, psychosexual counsellors and occupational therapists should take place within a multidisciplinary team, which should meet regularly: at least once a month.

Staff and training needs

Training in all aspects of urogynaecology (assessment, investigation, conservative and surgical treatments) is essential to ensure that best practice is taught. Training is provided through the RCOG subspecialty training or Advanced Training Skills Module programmes. The ATSM is an 'office urogynaecology' programme with 'basic' surgery, including assessment, investigations (including urodynamics) and primary surgery for urinary incontinence and prolapse. Subspecialty training allows the development of more clinical, surgical, analytical and research skills and experience in all aspects of urogynaecology. This development is important, as urinary incontinence and prolapse surgery are likely to become the most common procedures undertaken in gynaecology, following the introduction of medical treatments and conservative therapies for menorrhagia, infertility and cancer. Surgical competence is therefore important and NICE recommends a minimum number of procedures which should be undertaken to maintain skills. There should be at least 20 procedures of each operation for incontinence and/or prolapse performed per surgeon per year. NICE also recommends that incontinence surgery be performed by individuals working within a team

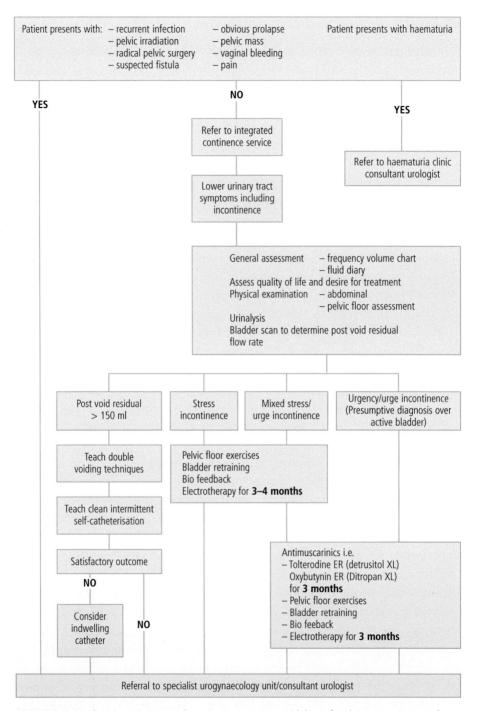

Figure 9.1 Southampton integrated continence service guidelines for the management of urinary symptoms in women (reproduced with permission)

where all aspects of the urogynaecological service are provided by appropriately trained individuals.

The British Society of Urogynaecology has suggested that 'one major case per working week per year' is necessary to maintain surgical competence (approximately 40 cases a year). At the present time, there is a question whether there is enough workload for all trainees and consultants to maintain their skills and so a training programme of more than 1 year might be required. However, this assessment of surgical competence based on numbers is in contrast to the educational recommendations of the RCOG, which focus on the acquisition, attainment and verification of surgical skills. It is possible that some individuals acquire surgical skills more rapidly than others and so demonstration of competence through objective structured assessment of technical skills might be more critical than performing a predetermined number of procedures. It is probable that both competency-based training and caseload are required to ensure surgical competence.

Of equal importance is the ability of a trainee to select appropriate patients for surgery. This requires regular outpatient work and discussion and review of cases at multidisciplinary team meetings.

Obstetrics will continue to be an important aspect of urogynaecology, especially in prevention of, for example, obstetric anal sphincter injury. It is recommended that individuals who undertake urogynaecological work should also be involved in labour-ward obstetrics to raise awareness and to provide teaching and training in pelvic floor dysfunction. Identifying women at risk antenatally might also be a useful role for the specialist urogynaecologist, so that preventative measures for incontinence and prolapse can be considered; for example, antenatal pelvic floor muscle training or, in selected cases, caesarean section (although the evidence for these as forms of prevention in the long term is as yet unclear).

Resource implications

As 'payment by results' and the new Healthcare Resource Group 4 codes for complex surgery evolve and become embedded in the NHS, it is likely that units which provide high-quality services by subspecialty and ATSM-trained urogynaecologists within multidisciplinary teams will attract more referrals and income. Implementation of the RCOG clinical standards and NICE guidelines are potential methods of ensuring 'high quality'. BSUG is therefore assessing the practicalities of introducing a system of accreditation of units to define and monitor standards of care, organisation and quality. They will 'recognise and badge' those units which comply with RCOG and NICE recommendations and this should not only promote best practice but also be attractive to primary care and NHS trusts in an ever-increasingly competitive 'market'.

Implementing the RCOG clinical standards, NICE guidelines and complying with the 18-week waiting time regulations will inevitably have resource implications. In addition, with the 18-week waits it is likely that women requiring follow-up appointments will experience long delays owing to a lack of capacity. Increasingly, other methods of follow-up, for example by specialist nurse or by telephone, might be required but auditing the outcome of these methods is essential. Additional resources for these changes and implementing evidence-based standards (including a patient-friendly and appropriate environment) will need to be identified on the strength of clinical governance and the adoption of the NHS 'quality care for all' paper.[17]

NICE has provided implementation advice for the urinary incontinence guideline.[2] Pelvic floor muscle training for women in a first pregnancy and the availability of sacral nerve root stimulation for intractable urge incontinence due to detrusor overactivity are recommended but how these are to be provided and funded has not been addressed. NICE suggests a possible solution: the financial savings made from the reduction in urodynamic investigations before surgery for 'pure' stress incontinence and the use of generic oxybutynin rather than more expensive alternatives might provide the necessary funding. However, it is questionable whether either of their recommendations has been implemented in clinical practice and if any such savings are used for implementing these specific guidelines.

Employing more physiotherapists and continence advisors should be a priority, which will likewise have resource implications. NICE has indicated that 'continence nurse advisers should be available in each health district. This role can be utilised as a resource within a supervisory, educational, coordination or clinical role in urinary incontinence services. Joined-up working across organisations may support more effective use of continence nurse advisers'.[18]

Audit and research

Patient-reported outcomes are strongly recommended for assessing the success of treatments. These measures allow clinicians to comply with

NICE recommendations, while providing personal data for their patients and they are also useful for appraisal and revalidation.

Data can be collected confidentially through the BSUG surgical audit database for urinary incontinence and prolapse, which provides validated instruments to assess outcome.[9] This database has the potential to provide national data on efficacy and safety for all incontinence and prolapse surgery.

Good-quality research is still required to answer many of the questions about surgical outcomes and, with the introduction of the UK comprehensive local research networks (CLRNs) it will become easier for clinicians to recruit patients to multicentre trials, through additional funding for local infrastructure. This should result in more rapid recruitment and trial completion. Local CLRNs should be contacted for further information. One example is a Health Technology Assessment Programme-funded multicentre trial of all prolapse surgery: PROSPECT (Prolapse Surgery, Pragmatic Evaluation by Randomised Controlled Trial), which will recruit up to 2500 women and should answer many of the questions about the outcomes of conventional prolapse surgery and newer procedures including vaginal mesh repairs.

References

1. National Health Service. 18 weeks: delivering the 18-week patient pathway [www.18weeks.nhs.uk].
2. National Collaborating Centre for Women's and Children's Health. *Urinary Incontinence: The Management of Urinary Incontinence in Women*. Clinical Guideline. London: RCOG Press; 2006 [www.nice.org.uk/CG040].
3. Robinson D, Anders K, Cardozo L, Bidmead J, Dixon A, Balmfoth J, Rufford J. What do women want? Interpretation of the concept of cure. *J Pelvic Med Surg* 2003;9:273–7.
4. Tincello DG, Alfirevic Z. Important clinical outcomes in urogynaecology: views of patients, nurses and medical staff. *Int Urogynecol J* 2002;13:96–8.
5. Hullfish KL, Bovbjerg VE, Gibson J, Steers WD. Patient-centered goals for pelvic floor dysfunction surgery: what is success, and is it achieved? *Am J Obstet Gynecol* 2002;187:88–92.
6. Rogers RG. The vexing problem of hidden incontinence. *N Engl J Med* 2006;354:1627–9.
7. Brubaker L, Shull R. EGGS for patient-centered outcomes. *Int Urogynecol J* 2005;16:171–3.
8. Srikrishna S, Robinson D, Cardozo L, Cartwright R. Experiences and expectations of women with urogenital prolapse: a quantitative and qualitative exploration. *BJOG* 2008;115:1362–8.
9. British Society of Urogynaecology. BSug.net database [www.bsug.net].

10. Scottish Intercollegiate Guidelines Network. *Management of Urinary Incontinence in Primary Care: A National Clinical Guideline*. SIGN Guideline No. 79. Edinburgh: SIGN; 2004 [www.sign.ac.uk/pdf/sign79.pdf].

11. National Institute for Health and Clinical Excellence. *Surgical Repair of Vaginal Wall Prolapse Using Mesh*. Interventional Procedure Guidance No. 267. London: NICE; 2008 [http://guidance.nice.org.uk/IPG267].

12. Jia X, Glazener C, Mowatt G, MacLennan G, Bain C, Fraser C, *et al*. Efficacy and safety of using mesh or grafts in surgery for anterior and/or posterior vaginal wall prolapse. *BJOG* 2008;115:1350–61.

13. International Continence Society [www.icsoffice.org].

14. International Urogynecological Association [www.iuga.org].

15. National Collaborating Centre for Acute Care. *Faecal Incontinence: The Management of Faecal Incontinence in Adults*. London: NCC-AC; 2007 [http://guidance.nice.org.uk/CG49].

16. International Consultation on Incontinence Modular Questionnaire (ICIQ). Bristol: Bristol Urological Institute; 2006 [www.iciq.net].

17. Department of Health. *High Quality Care for All: NHS Next Stage Review Final Report*. Cm7432. London: DH; 2008 [www.dh.gov.uk/en/Publicationsandstatistics/Publications/PublicationsPolicyAndGuidance/DH_085825].

18. Department of Health. *Health Outcome Indicators: Urinary Incontinence, Report of a Working Group to the Department of Health*. London: DH; 1999 [www.dh.gov.uk].

CHAPTER 10
Vulval disease

Charles Redman and Richard Todd

Key points

- ✓ Vulval disorders should be managed in the context of a specialist vulva clinic.
- ✓ A lead clinician with an interest and expertise in vulval disease should be responsible for running the clinic.
- ✓ Clinics should be easily accessible and be convenient for patients. Community-based clinics should be considered.
- ✓ Patient information should be readily available, both in the clinic and as a web-based resource.
- ✓ Clinics should be well equipped, ideally with a colposcope and couch and the facilities for biopsy.
- ✓ Clinics should be adequately staffed by appropriately trained individuals including a specialist gynaecology nurse.
- ✓ Management should be multidisciplinary with genitourinary consultants, dermatologists and chronic pain specialists. Access to psychosexual support should be available.
- ✓ Provision should be made to allow trainees access to the clinic.
- ✓ The lead clinician should be a member of a national or international vulval society and should attend educational meetings.
- ✓ Data from the clinic should be captured accurately and used in an audit programme which is presented to the multidisciplinary team at least annually.

Introduction

In the past, vulval conditions may have been seen by specialists lacking the necessary experience and knowledge to adequately assess, diagnose and manage such problems.

Often they would be seen in the context of a busy gynaecology, genitourinary or dermatology clinic lacking the resources, staffing and support structures necessary to ensure optimal care. As a result, some women may have found themselves misdiagnosed and given inappropriate or ineffective treatments. This suboptimal approach to care, although well intentioned, may have had consequences which were potentially harmful for the women concerned.

Although dedicated vulval clinics have existed in some units for many years, it is only relatively recently that the need for a structured, multidisciplinary approach to these problems has been recognised. The formation of a service to appropriately deal with vulval problems inevitably requires time, enthusiasm and resources. In a health service where competition for resources is intense, this presents its own challenges. With the advent of 'Choose and Book', the national electronic referral and booking service, patients now have a choice of where their care will be delivered. For those wishing to deliver vulval services, it is therefore vital that care of the highest quality is instituted and maintained.

The service user's view

Ideally, when planning services, you should draw upon information provided in patient surveys and questionnaires. In the case of vulval clinics, this information is lacking, although some parallels can be drawn with colposcopy services.

Vulval disease may be the subject of shame and embarrassment, with some women delaying seeking advice for months or years because of fears about the source of the condition or the examinations and investigations that may be necessary. There is good evidence that women have strong negative reactions to the intrusiveness of a gynaecological examination and women attending are likely to have high anxiety levels. It is therefore essential that a sensitive approach is taken and that every effort is made to put women at their ease and to protect their dignity.

Clinical standards and national guidelines

In June 2008, the RCOG published *Standards for Gynaecology*.[1] This document covers standards in gynaecological care in 20 key areas and has been subject to an extensive peer review process. These standards are to be used not only by healthcare professionals but also by commissioners, managers and providers. The ultimate objective of the document is to help provide an equitable and safe service with best possible outcomes for women seeking gynaecological care, as well as being of use in the quality assurance process.

Colposcopy has undoubtedly set a good example of how best to deal with these issues and many features of a colposcopy clinic transfer well to a vulval clinic.[2]

Clinics should be warm and should have a private area with changing facilities. Toilets should be readily available. Patients should be enabled to have a friend or relative present if they wish. If non-essential staff are present, such as medical students, this should be made clear and the woman should be given the option of whom she would like present at the consultation and examination. She should be given copies of correspondence if she requests them.

Model service outline and care pathways

Clinics should have clear clinical and operational guidelines. Usually, the lead clinician would be responsible for these guidelines. They should be written for the assessment of vulval conditions and algorithms drawn up for the management of the common vulval diseases.

The multidisciplinary team should aim to meet at least once a year, at which time the service can be reviewed, audits presented and planned and guidelines updated.

Figure 10.1 shows an example of a care pathway for benign vulval disease.

Patient information

Easily accessible patient information leaflets should be available in a range of languages to reflect the makeup of the local community. These leaflets should contain information on specific clinical conditions and the management options available. Clear information on the use of specific treatments, such as topical or systemic treatments, should be available. If possible, information about web-based resources should be given, as should contact details for patient support groups and forums.

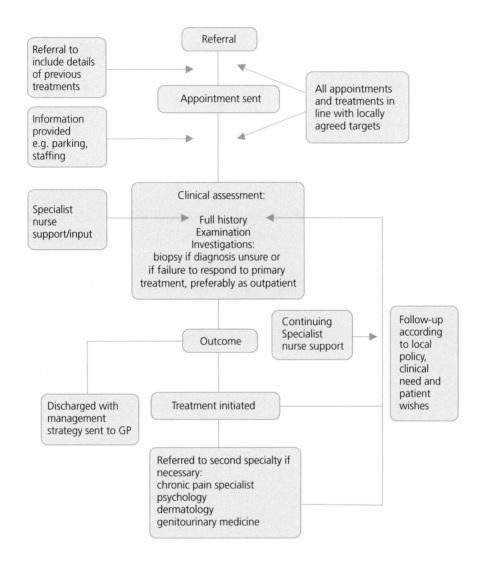

Figure 10.1 Example care pathway for benign vulval disease

Equipment

For adequate examination of the vulva, good access, lighting and magnification are a necessity. The use of a colposcope and couch is probably the easiest way to satisfy these requirements, although this is not strictly essential. Facilities should be available for photographic documentation of lesions and a video monitor is useful when demonstrating lesions to the woman if she wishes. Local anaesthesia and basic surgical instruments allow vulval biopsies to be performed if desired and haemostatic tools should be available under these circumstances. Resuscitation equipment must be readily available and staff appropriately trained in its use. The provision of computer equipment facilitates data collection and administration.

Resource implications

All women with suspected vulval problems should have prompt access to a clinic specialising in the management of such disorders. This would usually be hospital based but delivering care in a community setting may be more appropriate, depending on local needs. Systems should be in place to receive referrals from different sources, including primary and secondary care and these referrals should be seen in a timely fashion, in line with local targets. These targets need to be taken into account when planning clinics. Each clinic should have a named lead consultant and provisions should be made for a second clinician to provide cover in the event of leave. Timing of clinics should take the wishes and needs of patients into account. Ideally, there should be the option of evening appointments.

Staff and training implications

Crucial to the success of a vulval clinic is to have a named lead clinician with an interest and expertise in diseases of the lower genital tract. Although not essential, colposcopy accreditation is a valuable asset, owing to the multicentric nature of some conditions. Multidisciplinary support to the clinic is critical. Easy access to genitourinary medicine specialists, dermatologists and chronic pain specialists is vital. Psychosexual counselling services are also invaluable. In some settings, a combined clinic with these specialties may be possible.

As well as a healthcare assistant for each clinic room, each clinic should have a specialist nurse who is trained in the care of women with diseases of the lower genital tract. This nurse can act as a keyworker for the patient and provide a point of contact.

Administrative support should include a secretary with responsibility for the vulval clinic. Accurate data collection is important for the purposes of audit and quality control and an individual responsible for data entry should be identified.

Opportunities for specialist training

Unlike other aspects of gynaecology, such as family planning and colposcopy, no compulsory system of training and accreditation exists for the clinician treating vulval disorders. Whether this should change in the future is a matter for debate. The RCOG has, however, designed an Advanced Skills Training Module in vulval disease aimed at senior trainees in obstetrics and gynaecology. This module is designed to provide training in all aspects of vulval disease. It is also a component of knowledge for those doctors wishing to work in community based gynaecology or for those providing a gynaecological oncology service in the future. The multidisciplinary nature of the present service provision for women with vulval disease requires that trainees attend clinics in dermatology and genitourinary medicine as well as specialist vulval clinics.

Membership of a national or international society is encouraged. Both the British Society for the Study of Vulval Disease and the International Society for the Study of Vulvovaginal Disease hold annual meetings and core members of the multidisciplinary team should attend regular meetings.

Audit and research

To facilitate audit, a clinic pro forma which captures the required dataset should be designed. This can either be entered in real time if computer facilities allow or, alternatively, retrospectively by a data clerk. A programme of audits should be defined at the meeting of the multidisciplinary team and reviewed regularly.

Both clinical and non-clinical standards should be audited.[1] In particular, audits should take place of outcomes and responses to treatment, as well as complications of treatment. Patient satisfaction with the service should also be assessed on a regular basis.

References

1. Royal College of Obstetricians and Gynaecologists. *Standards for Gynaecology. Report of a Working Party.* London: RCOG; 2008 [www.rcog.org.uk/womens-health/clinical-guidance/standards-gynaecology].
2. NHS Cervical Screening Programme. *Colposcopy and Programme Management: Guidelines for the NHS Cervical Screening Programme.* NHSCSP Publication No 20. London: NHSCSP; 2004 [www.cancerscreening.nhs.uk/cervical/publications/nhscsp20.html].

Useful websites

British Society for the Study of Vulval Disease: www.bssvd.org
International Society for the Study of Vulvovaginal Disease: www.issvd.org

CHAPTER 11

Gynaecological oncology

Henry Kitchener and Andy Nordin

Key points

- ✓ The development of a national model of specialist teams and cancer networks has created high-quality equitable services across the country.
- ✓ Multidisciplinary team care is the core of cancer treatment.
- ✓ Patient-centred, evidence-based care is the central ethos of the service.
- ✓ The national cancer peer-review process provides an effective means of quality assurance to drive up standards and will evolve from assessment of process to that of outcomes, as effective tools for outcome measurement are established.
- ✓ Cancer waiting-time targets of 31 days from diagnosis to treatment and 62 days from referral to treatment have improved patient access.
- ✓ The role of the clinical nurse specialist is critical to support patients through the entire cancer journey.
- ✓ There is now adequate capacity for subspecialist training and accreditation, which are essential for the maintenance of a quality surgical oncology service and leadership of gynaecological oncology multidisciplinary teams.
- ✓ Audit is a necessary means of identifying deficiencies and improving quality.
- ✓ Research, particularly clinical trials, is critical to strengthening the evidence base and improving care.

Introduction

During the 1970s and 1980s, gynaecological surgeons with a special interest in oncology surgery established a number of services throughout Britain, mainly in university teaching hospitals. However, coverage of specialist gynaecological cancer care was patchy. Most women diagnosed with cervical, uterine, ovarian, vulval or vaginal cancer continued to be managed within small district general hospitals or teaching hospitals by generalist obstetricians and gynaecologists. As recently as the 1990s, the delivery of cancer care in general in the UK fell short of public expectation and was recognised as substandard. Survival rates were poor compared with those of the rest of Europe and the quality of care remained variable, with some highly specialised centres providing excellent care and others displaying a lack of specialised expertise. This persisting 'postcode lottery' became a national scandal.

The Government highlighted cancer services as an area of health care requiring modernisation, organisation and investment. An Expert Advisory Group to the Chief Medical Officers in England and Wales produced what was to become a seminal report on the direction of development of cancer services. The Calman Hine Report, *A Policy Framework for Commissioning Cancer Services*, was published in 1995 and laid out a national framework for the delivery of a properly organised and coordinated national cancer service.[1] It directed future development of services with a 'patient-centred' focus, aiming for equitable high-quality care across the country. The Calman Hine report called for the establishment of cancer networks, encompassing cancer units for diagnosis and management of common cancers in district general hospitals and specialist cancer centres to provide complex care and management of rarer cancers. The report called for establishment of multidisciplinary teams with designated lead clinicians, surgical subspecialisation and oncology-trained nurses, and the development of palliative care services.

The RCOG and the British Gynaecological Cancer Society (BGCS) responded to the Calman Hine Report in 1997 with a proposal for a series of gynaecological cancer centres managing a minimum of 200–250 cancers annually, serving a population of at least 0.75–1.0 million people, supporting the services of at least two subspecialist gynaecological oncologists.[2] Excepting specific low-risk cases of endometrial cancer, all gynaecological cancers would be referred from cancer units to cancer centres for treatment. To consolidate these proposals, the Department of Health commissioned a guidance document to formalise the model of care, as one of a series of documents for different tumour sites. The guidance document for gynaecological oncology was published in 1999. Commonly known as 'Improving Outcomes Guidance', this document has provided the framework for the reconfiguration of gynaecological oncology services in the United Kingdom.[3]

The NHS Cancer Plan was published in 2000, leading to the establishment of 34 cancer networks in England.[4] With its implementation, the last 10 years has seen a revolution in the delivery of gynaecological cancer care, ensuring greater equity of access, which will, it is hoped, also equate to improved and equitable outcomes.

The service user's view

One of the crucial elements of the Calman-Hine report was the need to place the patient at the centre of cancer care. This requires understanding and acknowledgement of the needs of the patient and her carers. As part of the National Surveys of NHS Patients programme, the Department of Health conducted a national survey to provide a benchmark of the quality of care provided by the NHS. The survey was carried out in 1999–2001 and referred to a period before the implementation of the Cancer Plan, involving over 65,000 patients drawn from over 170 NHS trusts. The only gynaecological malignancy covered by the survey was ovarian cancer, involving 3067 women. A further sample of patients was surveyed in 2004 by the National Audit Office to assess progress in patient experience following the implementation of the cancer modernisation agenda.

The provision of information regarding diagnosis and treatment options, in various forms (verbal, written and electronic), has become a cornerstone of gynaecological oncology services. The establishment of the role of the clinical nurse specialist has been key to this process. A core member of the multidisciplinary team, the clinical nurse specialist supports the gynaecological cancer patient throughout her cancer journey. In addition to providing emotional and practical support during the journey, the clinical nurse specialist provides assistance to patients to access resources and information from internet sites, patient support groups, charities and social services for domestic and financial assistance. We are now extending the context of the patient journey beyond treatment: the notion of 'survivorship'. Through investigating novel methods of cancer follow-up, the use of patient reported outcome measures, local and virtual (web-based) survivor support groups, targeted psychological and psychosexual support and other initiatives, we hope to assist women to make the transition from patient and cancer sufferer to survivor and provide them with appropriate assistance to manage long-term treatment related effects.

National guidelines and service standards

The 2005 National Audit Office publication, *Tackling Cancer: Improving the Patient Journey*, on behalf of the Department of Health, summarises the improvements made to the cancer patient experience in terms of waiting times, communication, information and other aspects of the quality of care.[5] While significant improvements had been achieved since the baseline survey, a number of other areas of concern were identified. These included deficiencies experienced by some patients in the areas of pain relief, psychological support, information regarding access to financial advice and complaints procedures, support for religious views and practices and frustrations from delays in appointments and investigations. The provision of palliative care services was highlighted as deficient in many parts of the country, limiting patients' access to hospice care and palliative care services at home and therefore restricting patients' end of life choices. This information was used to inform the cancer agenda, including peer-review guidelines and the Cancer Reform Strategy publication in 2007,[6] which directs the development of cancer services until 2012. In addition to the national audits, the views of patients and carers are integral to the function of cancer network gynaecology groups and local multidisciplinary teams. The peer-review process ensures that network groups include user representation and that clinical teams assess the views and experience of patients via patient support groups and audits.

The RCOG provides a complete set of standards for the provision of a streamlined service. The clinicians and commissioners should use these standards to develop national quality accounts.

Model service outline

In general, gynaecological cancers are diagnosed in cancer units or diagnostic localities in district general hospitals, by a gynaecologist who leads a 'rapid access' diagnostic service. Cancer units maintain a diagnostic multidisciplinary team meeting for review of pathology and imaging before referral to the local cancer centre. They provide low-risk endometrial cancer surgery but diagnostic localities feed all cases directly to the cancer centre. The cancer centre multidisciplinary team should ensure that appropriate diagnostic workup has been completed, usually involving specialised radiology and pathology review. It determines definitive management plans at various points on the patient pathway, based on agreed clinical guidelines which should be evidence based and regularly updated. Multidisciplinary team meetings are minuted, to provide an auditable record of decisions.

In certain cases, for example chemotherapy, the National Institute for Health and Clinical Excellence will recommend that certain regimens should be used in certain clinical settings. In many other instances, there are no national guidelines but evidence-based guidance should not vary a great deal between centres. The lack of national guidelines is being addressed by the Gynaecological Cancer Guidelines Group, which functions on behalf of the BGCS and the National Group of Gynaecological Network Leads to produce generic guidelines for the management of the main gynaecological malignancies.

Specialisation is at the heart of the multidisciplinary team, providing a high degree of collective expertise. This should ensure that consensus decisions are in line with expected national and international standards of care. The multidisciplinary team should also ensure that treatment planning is not idiosyncratic, nor dominated by a single clinician's views.

Training

The RCOG showed considerable foresight when it endorsed subspecialist training in the 1980s and adequate provision of subspecialty training posts now exists in the UK. Subspecialty training is based on a standard national curriculum which requires a minimum of 2 years of full-time clinical training and an additional major research component. Research in the field of gynaecological oncology is either performed as a separate entity (usually towards a higher degree) or the subspecialty training is extended to 3 years to include a significant component for research. The progress of trainees is carefully monitored and any concerns are required to be addressed in a timely fashion. Training should equip the gynaecological oncologist to undertake the full range of procedures which any given gynaecological cancer patient may require, but it is recognised that some of the most complex procedures will require surgical teamwork involving urologists, colorectal surgeons and plastic surgeons. As the patterns of disease and management change, so do the needs of trainees. For example, radical surgery for cancer of the cervix is less common than previously and the popularisation of laparoscopic surgery requires increased provision of appropriate training.

Audit

Quality assurance minimum standards of care in gynaecological oncology relate to the timeliness of treatment, the functionality of multidisciplinary teams and audits of various outcomes. The National Cancer Peer Review Programme is an integral part of the National Cancer Plan and the cancer modernisation agenda in England. Two cycles of peer review have been completed (2000–03 and 2004–07). Each involved intensive peer-review inspection of cancer networks and clinical teams, assessing configuration of services, infrastructure, clinical pathways and practices against a detailed set of standards or measures.[7] The peer review inspection reports are public documents and carry considerable weight within trusts and cancer networks. Deficiencies noted by the peer-review teams must be addressed as a matter of urgency, helping to drive up standards of care and creating an equitable service throughout the country.

Gynaecological clinical subgroups of the cancer networks oversee the standard of gynaecological cancer care across the network. This includes the implementation of clinical practice guidelines which form a benchmark against which audits can be performed. The guidelines are revised on a regular basis and all stakeholders must agree to implement them within their clinical teams. A clinical subgroup is required to undertake audits and this forms part of the peer-review process.

The introduction of cancer waiting-time targets was a theme of the National Cancer Plan. Patients with a suspicion of cancer must be seen in a specialist diagnostic clinic within 14 days of referral from primary care and definitive treatment has to begin within 62 days of referral and within 31 days of a firm cancer diagnosis being made. These targets have been rigorously monitored by the Department of Health, with trusts facing sanctions for breaches and, as a consequence, arrangements have had to be put in place whereby diagnostic workup and initiation of treatment are organised in an efficient manner.

To date, the quality-assurance agenda has focused on process rather than outcome. The Cancer Reform Strategy addressed this issue, with the establishment of the National Cancer Intelligence Network (NCIN), which will coordinate audits and routine measures of clinical outcome with data from the cancer registries. In collaboration with the NCIN, the BGCS and the National Group of Gynaecological Network Leads, the gynaecological oncology community is embarking on a national audit of surgical outcomes and complications. The UK Gynaecological Oncology Surgical Outcomes and Complications project will initially run as a web-based audit to collect robust baseline data of perioperative complications in gynaecological oncology surgery but it is hoped that it may be extended into routine clinical practice. It is anticipated that, shortly, survival and complications data for each gynaecological cancer centre will be readily available in the public domain, empowering patients to have confidence in their service provider.

Research

The era of molecular medicine in cancer has seen huge advances in our understanding of disease mechanisms and, as a result, targeted therapies are coming on stream at an increasing rate. To assess these and other innovative forms of treatment, the National Cancer Research Institute (NCRI) was established in 2001 to develop a portfolio of national trials. The NCRI Gynaecological Subgroup has been very successful in developing a portfolio of high-quality trials, including screening, medical and surgical treatment and follow-up. Trials are increasingly being performed as international collaborative studies and the results establish international standards of care. The appointment of National Cancer Research Network-funded research nurses to clinical teams throughout the country has enabled many teams to increase contribution to NCRI-adopted trials. Improving outcomes through clinical trials is incremental but, as well as determining how to improve survival, clinical trials have also shown us that we can achieve similar outcomes with less toxicity; for example, using doublet instead of triplet chemotherapy or using less radiotherapy.

References

1. Calman K, Hine D, Bullimore J, Davies T, Finlay I, Foster P, *et al. A Policy Framework for Commissioning Cancer Services. A report by the Expert Advisory Group on Cancers to the Chief Medical Officers of England and Wales.* London: HMSO; 1995.
2. Royal College of Obstetricians and Gynaecologists. *A Policy Framework for*

Commissioning Cancer Services. A Joint Working Group Response by the Royal College of Obstetricians and Gynaecologists and The British Gynaecological Cancer Society. London: RCOG Press; 1997.

3. NHS Executive. *Improving Outcomes in Gynaecological Cancers. Guidance on Commissioning Cancer Services. The Manual.* London: Department of Health; 1999 [www.dh.gov.uk/en/Publicationsandstatistics/Publications/PublicationsPolicyAndGui dance/DH_4005385].

4. National Health Service. *The NHS Cancer Plan: a Plan for Investment, a Plan for Reform.* London: DH; 2000 [www.dh.gov.uk/en/Publicationsandstatistics/ Publications/PublicationsPolicyAndGuidance/DH_4009609].

5. House of Commons Committee on Public Accounts. *Department of Health: Tackling Cancer: Improving the Patient Journey.* Nineteenth Report of Session 2005–06 Report, together with formal minutes, oral and written evidence. HC 790 Incorporating HC 485-i, Session 2004–05. London: The Stationery Office; 2006 [www.publications.parliament.uk/pa/cm200506/cmselect/cmpubacc/790/790.pdf].

6. Department of Health. *Cancer Reform Strategy.* London: DH; 2007 [www.dh.gov.uk/en/Publicationsandstatistics/Publications/PublicationsPolicyAnd Guidance/DH_081006].

7. NHS National Cancer Peer Review Programme. National Cancer Peer Review Measures: Gynaecological Oncology. Resources for Cancer Teams [www.cquins.nhs.uk/?menu=resources].

CHAPTER 12
Colposcopy services

Mahmood Shafi, Maggie Cruickshank and John Tidy

Key points

✓ Colposcopy has a well-developed training programme and commitment to continuing professional development.
✓ Quality assurance is given high priority and the whole service is subject to formal assessment on a regular basis.
✓ The training programmes were established over 10 years ago as a partnership between the British Society for Colposcopy and Cervical Pathology and the Royal College of Obstetricians and Gynaecologists, for medical or nursing qualified staff.
✓ Research and audit data are relevant in a national screening programme before the widespread introduction of new guidelines and technologies.
✓ The roll-out of liquid based cytology is now complete and data are awaited from other national initiatives that will inform the future screening and colposcopy services.

Introduction

Colposcopy services have been established in the UK since the 1960s, after colposcopy was introduced into clinical service by the early pioneers. Around that time, an *ad hoc* cervical screening service existed but it was not until 1988 that the programme was established nationally in a systematic manner under the auspices of the National Health Service Cancer Screening Programme (NHSCSP). The systemic approach has, to a large degree, underpinned the success of the screening programme, although latterly the service has been devolved to the individual countries (England, Wales, Scotland and Northern Ireland).

The national cervical screening programmes in the UK have led to high coverage of the at-risk population. For example, in England the NHSCSP currently achieves 78.6% coverage. There has been a gradual decline in the coverage rate (screened at least once in the previous 5 years) having been at a commendably high level of 82.5% in 1998.

There has been improvement in the provision of a rapid turnaround time for cervical cytology results and the aim is for all women to have communication within 2 weeks of the test being performed for screening purposes by 2010. Increasingly, direct referral systems are being established for abnormal cervical cytology to the colposcopy service. Recent guidance states that cervical cancers detected through the screening programme will be part of the Government's 62-day target for cancer treatment. This will require a rapid assessment of all high-grade (moderate dyskaryosis or worse) cytological abnormalities and it is suggested this should be within 2 weeks of the results being available. Those with lesser abnormalities currently are part of the 18-week referral-to-treatment targets and generally are seen within 5 weeks of the results being available.

The service user's view

Women being referred for colposcopy expect a rapid and professional service with sufficient information being provided in a format that is easily understood by them. The whole process of getting abnormal cervical cytology results, referral to colposcopy and possible treatment is associated with considerable stress (similar to that experienced before major gynaecological surgery) and appropriate information can be helpful in reducing these anxiety levels.

Clinical standards and national guidelines

Colposcopy was one of the early proponents of standards, both in relation to service and to training. The early standards documents were generally consensus based but informed by evidence. The first national guidelines were published in 1992, following a workshop convened by the National Coordinating Network. This has undergone several revisions and the latest version, *Colposcopy and Programme Management: Guidelines for the NHS Cervical Screening Programme*, was published in 2004.[1] This document forms the basis of colposcopy service provisions and standards relating to facilities and staffing.

NHSCSP guidance, and its equivalent in the other constituent countries of the UK, has led to the development of a high-standard colposcopy service in the UK. This has been facilitated by a quality assurance programme run regionally under the auspices of the cancer intelligence units. Each colposcopy unit is visited on a regular basis and national guidance is available in relation to the visiting programme that is coordinated by the NHSCSP Quality Assurance Group.[2] The visiting programme has powers of recommending service improvements with timelines. Progress against any recommendations can be monitored so that quality is uniformly of a high standard within the region. Quality assurance is monitored by Cervical Screening Wales and NHS Quality Improvement Scotland (NHSQIS) in Wales and Scotland, respectively.

Model service outline and care pathways

The NHSCSP[1] includes specific standards in relation to:

- screening programme policy
- screening strategies
- referral guidelines for colposcopy
- quality standards for colposcopy clinics
- diagnostic standards for colposcopy
- infections and colposcopy
- treatment of cervical intraepithelial neoplasia
- follow up of women attending for colposcopy
- pregnancy, contraception, menopause and hysterectomy
- screening and management of immunosuppressed women
- management of glandular abnormalities.

In addition to these standards, there is guidance on the working practices of colposcopy units. The service should be patient-focused, with written information provided in relation to the colposcopy and related procedures. Verbal advice should be available for women who request it. The colposcopy suite should be a dedicated facility, with changing areas and toilet availability. Counselling should take place in a private area before the woman changes for colposcopy.

During 2007–08, there were 122,000 referrals for colposcopy, with 80% of these being triggered by a screening test.[3] Of these, 30% were for moderate or severe dyskaryosis cytological abnormalities. Of those attending for the first time, 64% had some treatment or procedure at that attendance. Of those attending for high-grade cytological abnormalities, the proportion who had some treatment or procedure at that attendance was 84%. The most common procedure overall was a diagnostic biopsy, which was undertaken more often with low-grade cytological abnormalities. For those women attending with high-grade cytological abnormality, the most common procedure was an excisional treatment. The range of excision at the first attendance ranged from 16% in London to 61% in the East of England. For those women undergoing excision biopsies, 86% showed evidence of cervical intraepithelial neoplasia (CIN) or worse (range 83.8–90.2%).

Staff and training needs

The membership of the British Society for Colposcopy and Cervical Pathology (BSCCP) is around 2480, with 1600 certificated colposcopists. Of these, there are currently 190 certificated nurse colposcopists who undertake a significant caseload within colposcopy units. Certificated colposcopists are required to show continuing professional development and an audit of their activity, which is assessed every 3-year period in a recertification process. Each colposcopy unit should have a lead colposcopist, for whom a sample job description is available in NHSCSP guidelines.[1,4] The lead colposcopist needs to ensure good practice, compliance with protocols, data collection for mandatory KC65 returns (cervical screening statistics quarterly returns) and audit. A hospital-based programme coordinator is responsible for ensuring that quality-assurance targets are monitored, including non-attendance.

Clinic staffing requirements are detailed in NHSCSP guidelines, including advice in relation to nursing levels, administrative staff and secretarial support.[1] At all times, the clinic environment should protect the woman's dignity and women should have the opportunity to discuss their care both before and after the colposcopy examination or treatment. It is recommended that multidisciplinary team meetings should take place at least twice yearly, including cytopathology, histopathology and colposcopy staff, to discuss operational issues relevant to the colposcopy service.

The NHSCSP quality-assurance team wishes to extend personal audit for colposcopists to the following criteria but this is the subject of current discussion:

- number of new cases/year (standard more than 50 new cases referred with abnormal cytology)
- cytoreversion rates at 8 months after treatment (standard over 90% no dyskaryosis)
- confirmed histological treatment failures at 12 months (standard less than 5%)
- adequacy of biopsy for histology (standard over 90%)
- proportion of women treated at the first visit with CIN on histology (standard 90% or over).

Opportunities for specialist training

The BSCCP was one of the pioneers in setting down a training programme in conjunction with the RCOG. This programme was established in April 1998. Recently, a joint Advanced Training Skills Module (ATSM) has been developed for colposcopy, using the original format but revised to fit in with the RCOG's philosophy for ATSMs and to deliver a curriculum that is compliant with the goals of the Postgraduate Medical Education and Training Board (PMETB). This is now operative and individuals can register for training. The standards are the same whether the training is undertaken by a medically qualified practitioner or a nurse. All candidates need to register with the BSCCP before commencing their training and medically qualified practitioners may apply to undertake the programme at any stage in their training or in their post-training career. However, candidates who wish to complete an ATSM in colposcopy will have to apply via their training programme director before starting year 6 of specialty training. Competency is assessed through a variety of instruments developed by the College.

An objective structured clinical examination (OSCE) exit assessment has been developed to assess competency in a standardised situation. Performance is assessed by one or two examiners, using a structured marking sheet for a wide range of clinical and counselling skills. The training guide lists the domains (problems or conditions) with which the trainees should be familiar. The content of the OSCE covers a sample of these domains aligned with the learning outcomes and teaching methods of the curriculum. Blueprinting of the curriculum against relevant clinical skills ensures that a wide selection of relevant domains is covered, that the clinical content reflects reality and that there is a balance across them all.

The validity of the BSCCP OSCE has been assessed by an independent study to ensure that it meets PMETB recommendations. In particular, it has shown to be failing those candidates who should fail, providing for quality assurance of the assessment.

Resource implications

We currently have a well-developed ATSM for colposcopy, based on longstanding collaboration between the RCOG and BSCCP. Increasingly, nurses are undertaking colposcopy, diagnosis and treatment, with the ability to have dedicated teams working with consultant colposcopists. There has been support for this system from the nursing hierarchy and indeed from the employing hospital trusts. In the future, with human papillomavirus (HPV) vaccination being introduced, it is likely that fewer colposcopists would be needed but the impact of this vaccination will not be seen for many years.

Audit and research issues

HPV sentinel sites have been established in six laboratories nationally, following pilot studies. This addresses issues associated with introducing HPV testing into the cervical screening programme as triage for samples showing borderline nuclear change and mild dyskaryosis. The techniques of HPV testing and liquid-based cytology can be used together on the same sample without the woman having to be recalled for further testing. The HPV sentinel sites will additionally look at test of cure following treatment for CIN. Those women who would normally require annual cytology surveillance for 10 years may be discharged to a 3-yearly recall if both the cytology sample and HPV test are negative at the 6-month follow-up.

The TOMBOLA trial (Trial of management of borderline and other low-grade abnormal smears) addresses the issues of the most effective way to deal with women with borderline or mild smears. This trial has looked at the value of an HPV test to selecting management and the recommendations are based not only on detection and treatment of disease but also NHS and societal costs, rates of after-effects and complications and psychosocial issues.

The 'Artistic' trial (A randomised trial of HPV testing in primary cervical screening) is looking at the addition of HPV testing to cervical cytology screening. This will allow an estimate of the effectiveness of HPV as a stand-alone test and will determine the contribution of HPV detection to the cervical screening programme, as well as addressing methodological issues.

References

1. NHS Cervical Screening Programme. *Colposcopy and Programme Management: Guidelines for the NHS Cervical Screening Programme*. NHSCSP Publication No 20. London: NHSCSP; 2004 [www.cancerscreening.nhs.uk/cervical/publications/nhscsp20.html].
2. NHS Cervical Screening Programme. *Guidelines for Quality Assurance Visits in the Cervical Screening Programme*. NHSCSP publication No. 30. London: NHSCSP; 2008 [www.cancerscreening.nhs.uk/cervical/publications/nhscsp30.html].
3. NHS The Information Centre. Cervical Screening Programme, England 2007–08. [www.ic.nhs.uk/statistics-and-data-collections/screening/cervical-cancer/cervical-screening-programme-2007-08-%5Bns%5D].
4. Royal College of Obstetricians and Gynaecologists, British Society for Colposcopy and Cervical Pathology. *Standards for Service Provision in Colposcopy Services*. London: RCOG; 2006 [www.rcog.org.uk/womens-health/clinical-guidance/standards-service-provision-colposcopy-services].

CHAPTER 13
Laparoscopic surgery

Salma Kayani, Georgios Pandis, Alfred Cutner

Key points

Gynaecologists willing to set up a viable laparoscopic service need to:

✓ be familiar with the General Medical Council's guidance on consent
✓ be aware of the relevant RCOG guidance and clinical governance guidelines
✓ have satisfactory training and supervision before carrying out laparoscopic surgery independently
✓ undertake laparoscopic surgery where there is a facility of appropriate surgical equipment and supply of blood products
✓ put in place a coordinated system to deal with laparoscopic emergencies
✓ introduce and insist on a system of close postoperative monitoring
✓ demonstrate acute awareness of signs of postoperative complications
✓ audit their outcomes to help redesign and reconfigure the service
✓ understand that setting up a safe and effective service will enhance patient choice and improve outcomes.

Introduction

Gynaecological operative laparoscopy has progressed significantly over the past two decades. Initially, the routine application of endoscopic techniques only occurred for relatively straightforward procedures. However, advances in endoscopic equipment and the development of structured surgical training, combined with the acceptance of the advantages of laparoscopy, has led to the application of minimal access surgery in most areas of operative gynaecology.

Over 250,000 women undergo laparoscopic surgery in the UK each year.[1] Improving the standards of safety and surgical care is an essential principle in the establishment of new gynaecological services. The benefits of diagnostic and operative laparoscopic surgery in terms of reduced postoperative pain, shorter hospitalisation, earlier return to normal activities when compared with laparotomy, need to be balanced against the potential increased risks associated with minimal access surgery, such as vascular and organ damage. A 10-year report (1991–2000) from a major Australian medical defence organisation indicated that, although obstetric claims were more expensive, gynaecological claims were more frequent and operative laparoscopy was the second most common group of procedures involved in claims after hysterectomy.[2] Medical Defence Union (UK) data demonstrate that, over the past 10 years, it has opened 534 files with varying grades of claims regarding laparoscopic surgery.[3]

Since 2005, the National Health Service Litigation Authority (NHSLA) has dealt with 224 claims pertaining to laparoscopic surgery in gynaecology, of which 138 have resulted in damages paid.[4] Of these 224 claims, 204 have been for six most frequently occurring causes (Figure 13.1).The graph shows that the highest number of claims has been for intraoperative problems.

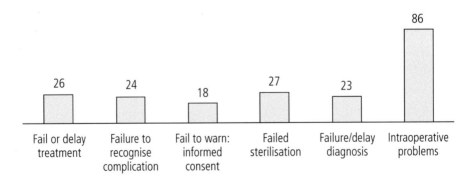

Figure 13.1 Six main causes of claims in gynaecological laparoscopy, 1 April 2005 to 31 October 2008 (n = 204) (NHSLA)

Women's expectations from laparoscopic surgery

Determining patient preferences and their direct or indirect involvement in the improvement of provision of health services is a legal duty of NHS organisations (section 242(1B) of the NHS Act 2006).[5] Eliciting patient preferences is part of the consent process for surgical procedures, where patients need to be aware of the risks and benefits of the operation and what alternative treatment modalities are available. Potential complications, such as vascular, visceral, bladder or ureteric injury should be discussed.[6] The difference between visceral injury and visceral surgery as part of the procedure should be clarified. For example, removal of a small part of bowel or bladder involved in disease such as endometriosis is part of surgical treatment and not a complication.

Laparoscopy is often referred to as 'keyhole' surgery, which may lead to confusion over the complexity of surgery and its associated risks. It is the surgeon's duty to dispel the myth that a 'small cut equals small operation' and ensure that the patient understands the true nature of the proposed intervention.

A postoperative discussion on the surgical findings, the course of recovery, including the use of images of the key elements of the procedure, is beneficial in the counselling process. Discussion of any adverse events or complications during surgery is vital to providing good patient care. As patients are discharged home shortly after having a laparoscopic procedure, there need to be mechanisms for contacting the hospital team if any complications arise.

Clinical standards and national guidelines

Laparoscopic surgery has progressed from a diagnostic to an operative tool. It should aim to emulate the open procedure. The RCOG, the National Institute for Health and Clinical Excellence (NICE) and the British Society for Gynaecological Endoscopy (BSGE) have produced clinical standards, benchmarks and national guidelines for the development, evolution and maintenance of units with laparoscopic facilities. NICE provides recommendations on the safety and efficacy of interventions, the RCOG produces guidance on the management of conditions and the BSGE is involved in the development of national benchmarks of skills and services.

Owing to the limited numbers of documents produced in the field of laparoscopic surgery, the RCOG has recently produced a working party report, *Standards for Gynaecology*, in which it has also recommended an outline on standards for laparoscopic surgery.[7] The following six main aspects of performance are included in this report:

- Women should be able to make informed choices about their care and management.
- There should be access to a suitably equipped laparoscopic theatre with high-quality video equipment.
- The process of laparoscopic surgery should be based on an appropriate risk management system that allows for improved quality of care. Regarding women with severe endometriosis, specialist referral centres should be developed.
- Outcome data on operators, procedures, entry techniques and complications should be prospectively audited.
- Staff training and maintenance of their competences should be at an agreed national level.
- Units performing laparoscopic surgery should adopt recommendations and guidelines from scientific bodies (RCOG, NICE, BSGE) and should benchmark their audited activity against the national standards.

The RCOG has provided guidance on consent for diagnostic laparoscopy,[8] preventing entry-related gynaecological laparoscopic injury,[9] the investigation and management of endometriosis,[10] the management of post-hysterectomy vaginal vault prolapse,[11] the management of tubal pregnancy[12] and the surgical treatment of urodynamic stress incontinence.[13] The RCOG guideline on vault prolapse highlights the requirement for a high level of laparoscopic skill and training for laparoscopic vault suspension.[11]

NICE has produced guidance on the following interventional procedures: total laparoscopic hysterectomy, laparoscopic supracervical hysterectomy, laparoscopic techniques for hysterectomy, laparoscopic laser myomectomy, laparoscopic radical hysterectomy for early stage cervical cancer, laparoscopic excision of pelvic lymph nodes, laparoscopic uterine cerclage, laparoscopic uterine nerve ablation for chronic pelvic pain and laparoscopic helium plasma coagulation for the treatment of endometriosis.[14]

Laparoscopic colposuspension is included in the NICE guidance on the management of urinary incontinence.[15] This guideline states that the open and laparoscopic procedures are equivalent. However, it does not recommend the laparoscopic route as a routine procedure, owing to potential cost implications and concerns over training. Thus, it is likely to become a specialist procedure performed by surgeons highly skilled in both continence care and laparoscopic techniques.

Finally, the General Medical Council[16] and the British Medical Association[17] have drawn up guidelines for the recording, copy, storage and transmission of medical images. Although it is accepted that medical images improve patient care, these images form part of the patient's medical record and require the same standard of confidentiality and the same requirement for consent to disclosure.

Model service outline and care pathways

Laparoscopic surgery requires teamwork not only in theatre but also throughout the patient journey. The patient's care begins once a referral has been received. In gynaecology, a multidisciplinary approach with 'named' members has mainly been a tenet of oncology services. Owing to increasing specialisation and multidisciplinary management of complex and chronic benign diseases, it has become an essential part of an effective approach to treatment in benign gynaecology. This approach is being driven in the management of severe endometriosis by the BSGE. Tertiary referral centres will be accredited to support training for advanced laparoscopic surgery for endometriosis. It is envisaged that such centres will be undertaking a minimum of 12 cases of severe disease each year. They will have a dedicated laparoscopic colorectal surgeon and will be required to submit patient data to a national database for audit purposes.

The main components for consideration when developing models of service in laparoscopic surgery are as follows.

Gynaecology outpatients

Systems should be in place to stratify referrals coming from various pathways (general practitioner, choose and book, secondary care and emergency admissions) to appropriate teams.

Multidisciplinary teams, including specialist nurses and healthcare professionals from other related specialties.

Development of specialist gynaecological ultrasound services enables women to be directly referred for diagnosis and management without the need to involve accident and emergency or general ultrasound services. This reduces duplication and provides an efficient service.

Assessment of patient satisfaction should be an integral component of any service evaluation.

Preoperative preparation

Detailed discussion complemented by written information on any diagnostic or therapeutic intervention.

Patient suitability for the laparoscopic approach should be determined, depending on relevant medical history.

Two-staged consent: first in clinic followed by confirmation on the day of surgery.

Liaison with the relevant associated specialist team.

Preoperative blood tests and bowel preparation.

Investigations as indicated.

Operative

Dedicated daycase and inpatient facilities are required with skilled staff, to enable efficient use of theatre time and appropriate support for women.

Anaesthesia staff familiar with laparoscopic surgery.

Local protocols for unexpected intraoperative complications such as bowel, bladder, ureteric or vessel injury.

Adherence to RCOG entry guidelines.

Postoperative

Follow enhanced recovery programme pathways, as recommended by the NHS Modernisation Agency.[18]

Ward staff familiar with the postoperative care of women who have undergone laparoscopic surgery.

Regular postoperative review of patients. Discuss operative details with patients. These may be supplemented with relevant images.

As patients who have undergone laparoscopy tend to go home earlier than those who have had laparotomy, provide a detailed information sheet covering what to expect during the recovery period in hospital and at home with contact details in case of an emergency.

Agreed protocols for management of postoperative complications.

A robust system whereby letters are sent to primary care concerning the operative procedure undertaken, discharge summary and intended follow-up.

Training in laparoscopic surgery

The challenge in complex excisional laparoscopic surgery is training and dissemination of operative technique in a safe and effective environment. Laparoscopic training can be developed and augmented with the use of simulators or laparoscopic trainers. The different methods of laparoscopic surgical training include box trainers, virtual reality training, live animal surgery and human cadaver training.

The safe practice of any surgical technique lies in effective structured training and supervised practice. The basic elements of this training are covered in the RCOG core training portfolio. For surgeons intending a career with a significant gynaecological surgical role, including intermediate level laparoscopic procedures, their training is covered by the Advanced Training Skills Module (ATSM) on benign gynaecological surgery, in which laparoscopy is an essential requirement.

For those surgeons intending to undertake complex laparoscopic procedures, this training will need to be supplemented by a process of mentorship, performing surgery of increasing complexity with the support of an experienced laparoscopic surgeon.[1] There is now an ATSM in advanced laparoscopic surgery which covers this area.

Learning and training is a lifelong process and hence consultants who have an interest in developing their minimal access surgery skills can identify colleagues with laparoscopic skills and make arrangements to enter into a preceptorship agreement to develop their skills.

Staff and resource implications

With the advancement of operative laparoscopy, there has been a responsibility to develop a parallel system that ensures accountability, quality of care, patient safety and best practice. For the entire system to perform optimally, it is important that surgeons are competent and that there is a harmonious evolution of staffing and resources are important.

Preoperative counselling to enable correct patient preparation and consent is vital in ensuring the best possible outcome. Only staff familiar with the surgery to be carried out should obtain consent.

Specialist nurses with a good knowledge of endoscopic surgery can be helpful in providing appropriate information, organising investigations, administering agreed drug therapies and offering psychological support to women. They can also run nurse-led clinics where the initial pre- or postoperative follow-up assessment can be carried out. When assessing the potential for laparoscopic surgery, the infrastructure and financial support of the institution to purchase equipment needs to be considered. However, sophisticated equipment without trained surgeons is of no benefit. Likewise, support staff to maintain and run the equipment is essential. Laparoscopic surgery necessitates a team approach between surgical, nursing and technical support staff.

The minimal access team need to be familiar with minimal access techniques and the technologies to be used. Regular in-house training sessions, attendance at national or international courses and meetings and, most importantly, dedication to the scope and activities of the laparoscopic team help consolidate and advance the service.

▨ Audit and research

Although intended to promote the ideal outcomes of better patient care and safety, the implementation of risk management may be costly and time consuming. The process requires committed leadership, appropriate provision of resources and dedication from all parties involved. For effective risk management in laparoscopic surgery, in addition to the guidance from the RCOG (where there is a trigger list for reporting in gynaecology),[9] the fundamental principles remain a stringent adherence to patient assessment and teamwork under the leadership of the senior surgeon.

Audit and research are fundamental to the development of an evidence-based approach and remain at the core of the development and natural progression of a modern service. Audit of length of stay, analgesia requirement, complication rate and readmission rate help to redesign and configure the service. This type of audit involves multidisciplinary team input, which focuses on the impact of teamwork on patient care.

Being a rapidly developing technology-based specialty, research on new technologies, their cost effectiveness and performance outcomes are important. Advances in laparoscopic surgery, such as three-dimensional cameras and robotics, require an active research programme.

Perhaps the future of laparoscopic gynaecology will be the

development of single-port surgery, which reduces the number of scars. However, this has to be counterbalanced by the size of the single incision and the impact on instrument manipulation. Industry is starting to drive this technology and its place has yet to be determined.

References

1. Royal College of Obstetricians and Gynaecologists. *Preventing Entry-related Gynaecological Laparoscopic Injuries.* Green-top Guideline No. 49. London: RCOG; 2008 [www.rcog.org.uk/womens-health/clinical-guidance/preventing-entry-related-gynaecological-laparoscopic-injuries-green-].
2. Singh SS, Condous G, Lam A. Primer on risk management for the gynaecological laparoscopist. *Best Pract Res Clin Obstet Gynaecol* 2007;21(4):675–90.
3. Claims analyses. *MDU Journal* 208;24(1):20–24.
4. National Health Service Litigation Authority. A report into claims in gynaecological laparoscopy. Personal communication. NHSLA, London. December 2008.
5. Department of Health. *Real Involvement: Working with People to Improve Health Services.* London: DH; 2008 [www.dh.gov.uk/en/Publicationsandstatistics/Publications/PublicationsPolicyAndGuidance/DH_089787].
6. Royal College of Obstetricians and Gynaecologists. *Obtaining Valid Consent.* Clinical Governance Advice No 6. London: RCOG; 2004.
7. Royal College of Obstetricians and Gynaecologists. *Standards for Gynaecology. Report of a Working Party.* London: RCOG; 2008 [www.rcog.org.uk/womens-health/clinical-guidance/standards-gynaecology].
8. Royal College of Obstetricians and Gynaecologists. *Diagnostic Laparoscopy.* Consent Advice No. 2. London: RCOG; 2008 [www.rcog.org.uk/diagnostic-laparoscopy].
9. Royal College of Obstetricians and Gynaecologists. *Preventing Entry-related Gynaecological Laparoscopic Injuries.* Green-top Guideline No. 49. London: RCOG; 2008 [[www.rcog.org.uk/womens-health/clinical-guidance/preventing-entry-related-gynaecological-laparoscopic-injuries-green-].
10. Royal College of Obstetricians and Gynaecologists. *The Investigation and Management of Endometriosis.* Green-top Guideline No.24. London: RCOG; 2006 [www.rcog.org.uk/womens-health/clinical-guidance/investigation-and-management-endometriosis-green-top-24].
11. Royal College of Obstetricians and Gynaecologists. *The Management of Post-hysterectomy Vaginal Vault Prolapse.* Green-top Guideline No. 46. London: RCOG; 2007 [www.rcog.org.uk/womens-health/clinical-guidance/management-post-hysterectomy-vaginal-vault-prolapse-green-top-46].
12. Royal College of Obstetricians and Gynaecologists. *The Management of Tubal Pregnancy.* Green-top Guideline No. 46. London: RCOG; 2004 [www.rcog.org.uk/womens-health/clinical-guidance/management-tubal-pregnancy-21-may-2004].
13. Royal College of Obstetricians and Gynaecologists. *Surgical Treatment of Urodynamic Stress Incontinence.* Green-top Guideline No. 35. London: RCOG; 2003 [www.rcog.org.uk/womens-health/clinical-guidance/surgical-treatment-urodynamic-stress-incontinence-green-top-35].
14. National Institute for Health and Clinical Excellence. Published interventional procedures [www.nice.org.uk/Guidance/IP/Published].

15. National Collaborating Centre for Women's and Children's Health. *Urinary Incontinence: The Management of Urinary Incontinence in Women*. Clinical Guideline. London: RCOG Press; 2006 [www.nice.org.uk/CG040].

16. General Medical Council. Making and using visual and audio recordings of patients. May 2002 [www.gmc-uk.org/guidance/current/library/making_audiovisual.asp].

17. British Medical Association Ethics Department. *Taking and Using Visual and Audio Images of Patients*. London: BMA; 2007 [www.bma.org.uk/ethics/confidentiality/AVrecordings.jsp].

18. Enhanced Recovery Programme, NHS Modernising Agency. Institute of innovation and achievement. (www.nodelaysachiever.nhs.uk)

CHAPTER 14

Gynaecological risk management

Leroy Edozien

Until recently, the management of safety in clinical practice was more informal than formal. Individual clinicians took steps to enhance the safety of their practice and a variety of quality improvement measures were in place at different times but there was no systematic approach to the understanding, measurement, monitoring and improvement of safety in clinical practice. Towards the end of the last millennium, a number of developments, including the emergence of clinical governance and the publication of *To err is human*[1] and *An organisation with a memory*,[2] brought about a major movement now known as 'patient safety'. The need to address an increasing burden of litigation also led to the concept of risk management in health care. Risk management is sometimes still perceived narrowly by clinicians as avoidance of litigation but it is more profitable to see it as a tool for enhancing patient safety, which is what it really is.

Risk management systematically identifies and evaluates factors that could expose patients, staff, visitors and hospital property to harm and puts in place defences which minimise the likelihood that such hazards will produce harm. The instinctive reaction of some clinicians would be that risk management is stifling but this should not be the case. On the contrary, and particularly when there is appropriate ownership, risk management empowers clinicians to use their skills and expertise in maintaining a safe healthcare environment.

Although obstetrics steals the limelight in risk discourse, gynaecology has its own share of patient safety incidents. Examples of these are given in Figure 14.1. As with other parts of the hospital, gynaecology departments should adopt a formal, systematic approach to managing

FAILURE IN DIAGNOSIS/TREATMENT

- Failure to diagnose:
  - cancer – ovarian, endometrial, cervical, vaginal
  - ectopic pregnancy
- Failure to exclude pelvic infection before hysterosalpingogram
- Failure to perform pregnancy test prior to sterilisation
- Latex allergy not addressed
- Failure to administer antibiotic or anti-thrombotic prophylaxis
- Failure to ensure biopsy specimen delivered to histopathology laboratory

DELAYED TREATMENT

- Delayed treatment resulting from alleged failure to action a change of address

UNNECESSARY PAIN

- Alleged negligent attempt to remove cervical polyp in clinic
- Failure to ensure appropriate disposal of fetal tissue

SURGERY WITHOUT VALID CONSENT

- Hysterectomy without consent
- Removal of both ovaries when only listed for removal of one or none

INTRAOPERATIVE PROBLEMS

- Damage to viscus during open or minimal access surgery
- Bladder, ureter, bowel, major blood vessel, uterine perforation
- Diathermy burns in peritoneal cavity, vagina or externally
- Wrong fallopian tube removed

INCOMPLETE/FAILED OPERATION

- Failure to remove both ovaries as planned during hysterectomy
- Unsuccessful surgical termination of pregnancy
- Incomplete evacuation of a miscarriage
- During sterilisation operation, contraceptive coil not removed
- Wrong cyst/mole/skin tag removed from vulva

FOREIGN BODIES RETAINED IN VAGINA OR ABDOMEN

- Wound drain, vaginal pack, swabs, surgical instruments, rubber tip of Spackmann's cannula

Figure 14.1 Some examples of patient safety incidents (extracted from the database of the NHS Litigation Authority)

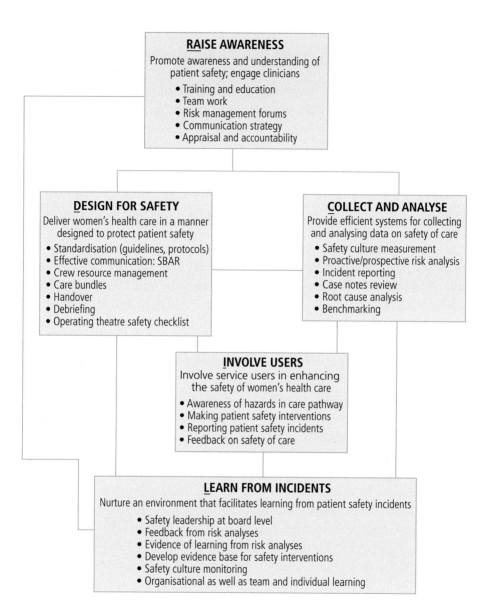

RAISE AWARENESS
Promote awareness and understanding of
patient safety; engage clinicians
- Training and education
- Team work
- Risk management forums
- Communication strategy
- Appraisal and accountability

DESIGN FOR SAFETY
Deliver women's health care in a manner
designed to protect patient safety
- Standardisation (guidelines, protocols)
- Effective communication: SBAR
- Crew resource management
- Care bundles
- Handover
- Debriefing
- Operating theatre safety checklist

COLLECT AND ANALYSE
Provide efficient systems for collecting
and analysing data on safety of care
- Safety culture measurement
- Proactive/prospective risk analysis
- Incident reporting
- Case notes review
- Root cause analysis
- Benchmarking

INVOLVE USERS
Involve service users in enhancing
the safety of women's health care
- Awareness of hazards in care pathway
- Making patient safety interventions
- Reporting patient safety incidents
- Feedback on safety of care

LEARN FROM INCIDENTS
Nurture an environment that facilitates learning from patient safety incidents
- Safety leadership at board level
- Feedback from risk analyses
- Evidence of learning from risk analyses
- Develop evidence base for safety interventions
- Safety culture monitoring
- Organisational as well as team and individual learning

Figure 14.2 The RADICAL framework for management of risk in health care

risk. One way of doing this is to adopt the RADICAL framework devised
by the author (Figure 14.2). This framework comprises the following key
steps:

- Raise awareness and understanding of patient safety
- Deliver women's health care in a manner designed to protect patient safety
- Involve service users in enhancing the safety of women's health care
- Collect and analyse data on safety of care, using efficient systems
- Learn from patient safety incidents; foster a learning environment.

Compliance and progress with this framework can be monitored by means of a checklist such as that in Figure 14.3.

Raise awareness and understanding of patient safety

Commitment to patient safety begins with awareness of the problem and understanding of the mechanisms underlying clinical error.[3] Awareness of the problem of patient safety has grown in the last decade but understanding of the epidemiology remains less than satisfactory. A full discussion of the psychology of human error is beyond the scope of this chapter but it is important for clinicians to grasp basic concepts such as situational awareness, defences and latent and active factors in medical accidents.[4] When we understand how errors happen, we can begin to identify error-producing conditions in our pathways of care. These conditions may be regarded as latent pathogens waiting to strike once vulnerability is exposed.

The clinician whose unsafe act or error led to the accident is at the sharp end of things but they may have been left vulnerable by deficiencies at the organisational level in areas such as service design, workforce planning, procurement of equipment, policies and strategies. Apart from their own knowledge, competence and confidence, the individual's vulnerability may have been enhanced by contributory factors such as patient attributes (for example, obesity increasing the risk of complications in laparoscopy), task factors (such as the use of a sharp trocar for a blind entry into the peritoneal cavity), team factors (for instance, the availability of supervision or support from an experienced laparoscopist), environmental factors (such as the availability of appropriate equipment for laparoscopic surgery) or organisational factors (for example, a poor safety culture meant that there was poor supervision or lack of investment in equipment). Patient safety incidents often happen because of the clinician's loss of situational awareness (their cognitive appraisal of what is happening differs from reality). For example, they are unaware

Raise awareness and understanding
- Simulation/scenario training is undertaken regularly in our unit
- We have a communication strategy for disseminating patient safety information (through ward meetings, newsletters, departmental meeting, notice-boards, etc.)
- Risk management is an important element in the induction of new staff and appraisal and of all staff
- Risk management is a key feature of our educational meetings
- We continually measure our safety culture using validated tools for doing this

Design for safety
- Our unit has evidence-based guidelines and protocols for all common clinical conditions
- We have implemented bundles of care for selected clinical conditions
- We have formal policies for handover of care and these are audited periodically
- The use of a perioperative safety checklist is in place and this is audited periodically
- Our staff have formal training on communication tools such as SBAR and Readback.

Involve users
- Our patients are actively encouraged to report safety incidents and these are logged in our incident reporting system
- Our patients are encouraged, through information leaflets and other means, to make or initiate safety interventions
- User involvement is a standing item in our clinical governance committee meetings
- Our patient information leaflets include information which could help reduce the risk of patient safety incidents
- We periodically give feedback to our patients on the safety of the care we provide

Collect and analyse safety data
- We have an incident reporting system and it is used by all cadres of staff
- Risk assessment is prospectively conducted in all clinical areas
- The department has a risk register and major risks are escalated to the hospital-wide register
- System analysis (root cause analysis) is conducted for major incidents and a database of these analyses is maintained
- We have up-to-date data on the safety of the care we provide and can compare our performance with standards elsewhere

Learn from patient safety incidents
- In our unit, specific targets have been set for selected patient safety indicators (e.g. in relation to surgical site infection)
- The findings of every root cause analysis have been widely disseminated and action plans have been implemented
- It is clear to our staff that the trust board prioritises patient safety
- Safety culture assessment shows that we have the attributes of a learning organisation
- Our risk management, complaints and claims handling systems talk to each other

Figure 14.3 Checklist for implementation of RADICAL risk management standards

that the structure they are about to clip is not a fallopian tube but a round ligament or, because their focus is on another structure, they are unaware that a loop of bowel is about to come in contact with the diathermy forceps. This may be associated with inattention, fatigue, stress, reduced working memory capacity, poor communication, undue workload or working to meet tight deadlines or schedules. Sometimes incidents happen because of violations of or deviations from standard operating procedures.

Unless clinicians and managers understand the underlying mechanisms and the consequences for patients, they are unlikely to be motivated to make the necessary changes or take the correct approach.

Design for safety: deliver health care in a manner designed to protect patient safety

Human error cannot be totally eliminated but the risk of patient safety incidents can be reduced if, at individual and unit levels, we aim to provide care in a way that reflects safety awareness and a commitment to reducing the likelihood of error. This means paying attention to things like communication, consent, confidentiality, training and supervision and provision of patient-centred care. It also means looking at what could go wrong in clinical areas, such as the outpatient clinic and operating theatre, and putting defences in place.

Guidelines, standards and clinical audit

Staff should have access to referenced, evidence-based multidisciplinary guidelines for the management of common gynaecological conditions. Guidelines, protocols and policies should be reviewed and updated when there has been a major change in the evidence base or according to a schedule specified on the document but no later than every 3 years. Adherence to guidelines and protocols should be monitored by criterion-based clinical audit.

Consent

All patients undergoing treatment should be given appropriate information on the nature and purpose of the treatment, benefits, alternatives and risks and the consent process must comply with the hospital's consent policy. The emphasis here is on consent as a process, not merely obtaining the patient's signature on a consent form. The idea that consent is not an end in itself but a means to responsible participation by patients in their own care and a means to a mutually rewarding relationship between clinician and patient is one that needs to be more widely promoted among gynaecologists.

Handover of care

Handover is a weak link in the process of care; without active management this process readily predisposes to or precipitates patient safety incidents but, with implementation of a simple handover protocol, errors can be reduced with little or no cost in time and resources.[5] It is not uncommon for a woman admitted as a gynaecological emergency to remain on the ward without being seen by a doctor or without a clear plan of action or to have her treatment delayed as a result of inadequate handover. Patients have died as a result of this kind of lamentable lapse. There should be a personal (and, if possible, recorded) handover of care between staff when there is a change of shift and when a patient is transferred from one professional to another.

Governance structures and processes should also address issues such as training and supervision, reduction of surgical site infection and introduction of new service models, techniques and technology.

Involve service users in enhancing the safety of health care

As with other aspects of care, risk management calls for partnership with patients: there should be no talk of patient safety without patients. Patients can be engaged in a variety of ways: keeping them informed of policies, initiatives and statistics, involving them in the design or reconfiguration of services to enhance safety and in the protection of their own safety (for example, by avoiding misidentification).[6]

Collect and analyse data on safety of care

To improve safety in the care we deliver, we must know the current rates of patient safety incidents in our practice and then we must have structures and procedures for monitoring our progress on the road to safer care. This is not always as easy as it sounds. Patient safety science is still a relatively new field in health services, so appropriate metrics are often not available or staff are not familiar with them. This is a field where human behaviour is a dominant confounder and one that is often difficult to predict, assess and control. It is not enough merely to collect incident reports and amass huge amounts of data on patient safety incidents. For such data to be meaningful, they have to be analysed and used constructively to change practice where necessary and demonstrate safer care. The raw data have to be converted to information which is meaningful and of practical benefit to staff and service users. Finally, there is no one size that fits all and each unit will have to adapt the general principles described here to its own circumstances.

Learn from patient safety incidents

Organisational learning is an important element in risk management. It is bad enough to have patient safety incidents; to fail to learn from them runs counter to our professional ethics. Organisational learning, however, is not a passive osmotic process; it has to be actively promoted and the learning environment has to be nurtured. In the context of patient safety, a learning organisation is one that is able to create new knowledge from patient safety incidents, learn from its experience and that of others, transfer knowledge acquired and bring about change in its behaviour as a response to the new knowledge.

Individuals taking responsibility

While it is important that gynaecology departments, as organisational units, should have structures and processes in place to manage risk, it is also important that individual gynaecologists should incorporate the principles of risk management in their clinical practice. Taking a systems approach is important but it is just as important to hold individuals accountable for their practice. The management of risk within the unit or team is not just that of the risk lead or the risk management committee. The role of the risk lead is not to manage everyone's risk but to facilitate the efforts of clinicians and support workers in managing risks in their own practice.

Although it may be fashionable to speak of a 'no-blame culture' and to over-emphasise the role of systemic pathogens in the aetiology of patient safety incidents, it is more appropriate to speak of a 'fair (or open) culture' and to find the right balance between both the 'system' and the 'person' approach. This is partly because some incidents result from the clinician's outright violation of established best practice. Perhaps more importantly, the individual at the sharp end offers the last line of defence against an accident and it helps if the individual is aware of this responsibility. It may be that specialist recertification will induce clinicians to pay more attention to this responsibility.

Research

As with other aspects of clinical practice, interventions to promote patient safety should be supported by evidence. Unfortunately the evidence is often either absent or thin and clinicians brought up on a diet of 'evidence-based medicine' may have little or no confidence in these interventions. It is important both for the direct benefit of patients and for the engagement of clinicians that research into best practice in the management of healthcare risk should be promoted. While significant strides have been made in patient safety research in anaesthesia and general surgery, relatively little has been done in women's health. Possible research questions cover a wide range of issues, including how to deal with problems of the learning curve,[7] the efficacy of interventions to engage patients in patient safety,[8] the appropriate indicators for measuring safety in gynaecology, the risk implications of evolving trends in care (such as increased use of medical management of ectopic pregnancy[9]) and the relationship between surgical volume and complication rates[10].

Conclusion

Models of care in women's health, whether addressing generalist or specialised care, should incorporate the management of risk. Safety is inseparable from quality of care and there are statutory and professional obligations to provide good-quality care. The commitment to patient safety applies at organisational as well as individual level, and is operational through risk management structures and processes. The RADICAL framework provides a convenient vehicle for implementing and monitoring risk management.

Acknowledgement

The NHS Litigation Authority kindly made available the database from which Figure 14.1 was produced.

References

1. Committee on Quality of Health Care in America. *To Err Is Human: Building a Safer Health System.* Washington DC: National Academy Press; 2000.
2. Department of Health. *An Organisation with a Memory: Report of an Expert Advisory Group on Learning from Adverse Events in the NHS.* London: The Stationery Office; 2000.
3. Weingart SN, Wilson RM, Gibberd RW, Harrison B. Epidemiology of medical error. *BMJ* 2000;320:774–7. DOI: 10.1136/bmj.320.7237.774.
4. Reason JT. Understanding adverse events: the human factor. In: Vincent C, editor. *Clinical Risk Management: Enhancing Patient Safety.* 2nd ed. London: BMJ Books; 2001. p.9–30.
5. Catchpole KR, de Leval MR, McEwan A, Pigott N, Elliott MJ, McQuillan A, *et al.* Patient handover from surgery to intensive care: using Formula 1 pit-stop and aviation models to improve safety and quality. *Paediatr Anaesth* 2007;17:470–8.
6. Entwistle VA, Ian S. Watt IS. Patient involvement in treatment decision-making: the case for a broader conceptual framework. *Patient Educ Couns* 2006;63:268–78. DOI: 10.1016/j.pec.2006.05.002.
7. Healey P, Samanta J. When does the 'learning curve' of innovative interventions become questionable practice? *Eur J Vasc Endovasc Surg* 2008;36:253–7.
8. Davis RE, Jacklin R, Sevdalis N, Vincent CA. Patient involvement in patient safety: what factors influence patient participation and engagement? *Health Expect* 2007;10:259–67.
9. Edozien LC. Medical gynaecology comes full circle: the management of ectopic pregnancy from Tait to date. In: Hillard T, editor. *Yearbook of Obstetrics and Gynaecology Volume 12.* London; RCOG Press; 2007. p. 15–33.
10. Hanstede MM, Emanuel MH, Stewart EA. Outcomes for abdominal myomectomies among high-volume surgeons. *J Reprod Med* 2008;53:941–6.

CHAPTER 15

The role of the clinical director

Gavin MacNab

Key points

- ✓ Effective communication is a key role for the clinical director.
- ✓ Leadership is about developing teams, managing teams, monitoring progress and acknowledging success.
- ✓ Sell the RCOG standards for gynaecology enthusiastically and with conviction.
- ✓ Be prepared to carry out developmental work, such as team building, if required.
- ✓ Identify lead for all the standards.
- ✓ Provide support in terms of time and personnel appropriate for achieving implementation.
- ✓ Develop reporting framework and agreement from lead consultants.
- ✓ Monitor progress regularly throughout the year.
- ✓ Produce an annual report and circulate this widely.

Introduction

There are understandable anxieties that this document becomes another quick read and is then consigned to that dusty pile of papers in the corner of the office never to see the light of day again.

Clinical directors may feel a reluctance to tackle standards for gynaecology, as implementation will require additional work within a climate of fatigue and burnout following years of Department of Health-driven targets and implementation of national service frameworks, National Institute for Health and Clinical Excellence guidance, Clinical Negligence Scheme for Trusts/NHS Litigation Authority (CNST/NHSLA) standards, NHS Quality improvement standards reviews in Scotland, cancer peer reviews, Human Fertilisation and Embryology Authority visits, Colposcopy Quality Assurance Review Centre visits and on and on.

A cursory glance at the *Standards for Gynaecology* document[1] may leave the impression that there is not much work to be done. A more detailed read exposes deficiencies in services. In our department, gynaecology guidelines and patient information has lagged behind obstetrics. I suspect that this has occurred because there have not been the incentives that litigation concerns and CNST/NHSLA work has brought to bear on obstetric practice.

Clinical directors should view the *Standards for Gynaecology* as the opportunity to convince the RCOG that we, not the College Tutors or the Regional Advisers, are the key to raising standards in obstetrics and gynaecology. Furthermore, the document also gives us an unprecedented opportunity to identify gaps in our service provision and to develop an informed business case for seeking additional funding from the strategic health authorities.

I am convinced that implementation of RCOG standards will only take place with the support of the clinical directors. After all, one of our key responsibilities is to deliver high-quality services.

The themes in *Standards for Gynaecology* are surely ones that we can all relate to and feel passionately about, namely:

- access to services
- patient information
- the environment in which services are delivered
- practice of evidence-based guidelines
- audit and continuous improvement
- risk management in a culture of shared learning
- adequate training for all staff.

It seems highly likely that attention to all these themes will deliver a high-quality service. Successful implementation of these standards will require a multidisciplinary team approach but consultant colleagues, as always, will be critical in terms of leadership.

Complying with these standards may prove easier for larger units than for smaller ones. However, no unit should exempt themselves from the task ahead otherwise the RCOG will fail in its mission of 'setting standards to improve care of women' to develop equitable, safe and high-quality services for all women. We must ensure safe delivery of service, delivered by experienced doctors, fit for purpose, as we believe that such environments will be conducive to delivering high-quality training for doctors in training as well.

Management systems vary between trusts and there will be no 'One fix fits all' approach to tackling standards in gynaecology. There are, however, key roles and responsibilities that will apply to all clinical directors if the Royal College of Obstetricians and Gynaecologists vision is to be realised.

Key roles and responsibilities of clinical director

- Communication
- Leadership and team building
- Vision
- Facilitation and support
- Production of a reporting framework
- Production of an annual report
- Identification of leads
- Developing a reporting timetable

Communication

Clinical directors are viewed as the interface between the department and the trust executive board, other specialties, primary care trusts and commissioners of services. Effective communication, both externally and within the department, is a key role and responsibility for a clinical director.

There are many different styles and methods of communication. The essential message that must go out to staff from clerical and administration to consultants is that all make themselves aware of the RCOG standards and the clinical director's commitment to achieving those standards.

Leadership and team building

A clinical director will struggle to implement standards if they are not in charge of a functional team of consultants and all other staff who contribute to providing high-quality services. If the team is not pulling together the RCOG standards may act as a catalyst. In addition, it is important that these issues are allocated enough time for discussion and for team building purposes.

Leadership is about developing teams, managing teams, monitoring progress and acknowledging success. As with risk management, the functionality of the whole team will be the most crucial determinant of success or failure of implementation of *Standards for Gynaecology*.

The RCOG vision

The clinical director has a vital role in selling the RCOG vision with zeal and determination. Any negativity will be seized upon by some or all of the team as the excuse 'to sit tight and do nothing'. Determination to see the job through can inspire the team but will probably not be enough on its own. It may be useful to use one of the standards to demonstrate what you hope to achieve. There may be a standard in which there are glaring deficiencies at a local level. An example might be services for termination of pregnancy which may have been allowed to drift to an alternative provider because of more pressing priorities. The standard is that there are many different successful models. The ideal service, however, has a consultant lead with close links to primary care, provision of contraceptive and sexual health care, counselling and gynaecology services. A high-quality service will require a lead consultant in gynaecology to be involved and probably leading the service if no other suitably qualified consultant is available.

Each clinical director will know the best approach to selling a vision. It is an important phase of the project and failure to win over hearts and minds at an early stage may jeopardise successful implementation.

Facilitation and support

The clinical director must demonstrate their commitment and support for the implementation process. Allocation of time within the job plans of a lead consultant demonstrates support but also places a greater obligation on the individual consultant to deliver what is required. It may be necessary to offer advice in areas such as guidelines, patient information and audit. The provision of secretarial support is always gladly received and may be essential in achieving the objectives.

When looking at the standards, I was struck by the vast array of connections with other services within and outside the trust. These vary from child protection issues, NHS Direct/NHS 24, interpreter services, sexual health services and psychosexual medicine, to name but a few. The clinical director must ensure that these connections are in place or can be put in place to avoid frustration or demotivation at lead consultant level. This again emphasises the key communication role for the clinical director.

Clinical audit and outcome indicators

It will be prudent to build a unit strategy for outcome indicators for individual services, as described in this document, which would not only provide data for service quality improvement but would also support recertification of doctors in the future. It is important to invest in developing a high-quality information system which could also collect clinical risk management data related to individual service.

Reporting framework

Understanding the RCOG vision is extremely important and much preparatory work must be carried out by the clinical director before this can be achieved. The first question is likely to be 'How is this going to happen and how much work does it mean for me?'.

The framework should be uniform for all standards and may include the following aspects.

Identification of a lead consultant and members of the governance group, with specialty trainee and lay person involvement.

Description of the patient care pathway taking account of local needs.

A detailed report on compliance and noncompliance against each item within the standard, together with an action and nominated responsibility for each action plan.

Evidence of new guidelines.

Evidence of audit and change in practice.

Governance meetings held at least 6-monthly, with minutes.

Finally, the lead clinician should develop a 'road map' beyond the RCOG standards, to avoid a static state and complacency.

Annual report

All the work carried out over a 12-month period can be compiled into an annual report, measuring performance against each standard and also benchmarking the unit's performances against the previous year's data. This will demonstrate the clinical director's determination to complete the task and also creates a culture of competition among contributors, which is usually healthy.

The annual report will be useful in terms of identifying progress towards the standards. It can also be shared with the trust clinical governance steering group, executive board, commissioners of services and even the general public.

There should be a clear statement about any deficiencies in services which need to be addressed. The management always likes to see a solution for the questions raised in the report to satisfy non-executive directors of the trust board that solutions are being developed to meet the gaps in the service.

Identification of leads

There are 20 standards for gynaecology. There will be very few units which are large enough to identify individual consultant leads for each standard. Some degree of grouping of the standards will be required and this will vary from trust to trust. I can demonstrate this by sharing with you my plans for tackling *Standards for Gynaecology* (Table 15.1). With this kind of grouping, it only requires six consultants and the risk manager to incorporate all 20 standards.

Reporting timetable

The reporting framework and reporting timetable should be shared with consultant leads one year in advance of production of an annual report.

Month one

Lead consultant checks standards using the reporting framework and identifies compliance or noncompliance against all items within the standard. Where there is noncompliance, the lead produces an action plan with nominated responsibility and a provisional timescale for

Table 15.1 A plan for tackling standards for gynaecology

Standard	Topic	Lead	Notes
1	Generic standards for the provision of gynaecology services	Clinical director	This would be appropriate for any clinical director
19	Organisation of outpatient clinics		
2	Early pregnancy loss	Consultant A	One of our obstetric consultant leads has an interest in both the obstetric care of women with recurrent miscarriages and early pregnancy loss
3	Ectopic pregnancy		
4	Recurrent miscarriage		
5	Infertility	Consultant B	Lead consultant for reproductive medicine also shares a gynaecology/endocrine clinic with an endocrinology physician
12	Menopause		
6	Pelvic inflammatory disease	Consultant C	Genitourinary medicine consultant (fortunately, genitourinary medicine is part of our directorate)
7	Termination of pregnancy	Consultant D	One consultant has subspecialty training in contraceptive services
8	Female and male sterilisation		
9	Diagnostic and operative hysteroscopy		
10	Laparoscopic surgery	Consultant E	One consultant has an interest in all three areas
13	Urogynaecology		
11	Heavy menstrual bleeding		
14	Benign vulval disease	Clinical director	Clinical director is also unit cancer lead
15	Colposcopy		
16	Gynaecological oncology		
17	Risk management	Risk manager	We have two risk manager midwives but one of these oversees gynaecology issues as well
18	Gynaecological examination		
20	Record keeping in gynaecology		

completion of the task. At the same time, an attempt should be made to draw up a patient care pathway to highlight any significant gaps in the service.

Month two

Lead consultant meets with clinical director (allocate sufficient time) to discuss the review against standards. At this point, some prioritisation may be necessary. If, for example, guidelines are in a rudimentary phase then some degree of selection may be required in the first year. The clinical director and lead then agree the tasks to be completed in the first year.

Month four

Lead consultant meets with clinical director to discuss progress against action plans. Clinical director checks evidence of early work, such as description of patient care pathway, new guidelines, audit projects and medical trainee involvement.

Month eight

Lead consultant meets with clinical director to discuss progress and a reminder is given about the submission date for the final report on work carried out in that year.

Month ten

All submissions should have been received by clinical director.

Month twelve

Clinical director produces the annual report detailing progress towards achieving the RCOG's standards for gynaecology. This report can be submitted to the trust clinical governance steering group, the executive board and others.

This seems an exhausting process but the workload for all will decline steeply in the following years if compliance against standards is achieved and maintained.

How to take forward your quality agenda

Once the directorate team has completed its yearly report, this should be widely shared within the department. It is important for all colleagues (consultants and medical managers) to discuss these findings, identify service gaps and prioritise key objectives for service improvement. The key findings from this report should be fed back to management, with appropriate costing models clearly demonstrating efficiency, service improvement and how clinical governance issues would be addressed.

Reference

1. Royal College of Obstetricians and Gynaecologists. *Standards for Gynaecology. Report of a Working Party*. London: RCOG; 2008 [www.rcog.org.uk/womens-health/clinical-guidance/standards-gynaecology].

CHAPTER 16
Recommendations

Tahir Mahmood, Allan Templeton nd Charnjit Dhillon

The RCOG published its document *Standards for Gynaecology* in 2008 and is being used widely by commissioners, providers and policy makers. It sets out the principles of quality assured gynaecological services. This section has identified some key indicators as exemplars, although we recommend that you make use of the whole document.

Gynaecological services: generic

- For women attending a one-stop clinic, the pre-appointment letter for clinic attendance should provide clear information regarding the procedure and investigations that might be performed.
- Treatment and care should take into account women's individual needs and preferences.[1]
- There should be clear verbal and written information on all aspects of treatment available.
- There should be a clear pathway for referral to local child protection teams, including the management of young people under the age of 13 years who are sexually active.
- A policy should be in place to support and refer potential victims of domestic and sexual abuse.
- There must be a designated reception area, staffed with an appropriately trained receptionist.
- A clearly defined pathway for relevant investigations and referral arrangements should be in place.
- All units should have written advice for training-grade doctors on when to seek help and what procedures they may perform without direct supervision.
- Robust arrangements must be in place to ensure that locum, bank or

agency staff receive an appropriate induction and are competent to perform their duties, and that they are provided with guidance in the form of a locum pack.

Early pregnancy loss

- Women should be offered a range of management options with a full explanation of the processes involved.
- All emotional and psychological counselling requirements should be provided within the early pregnancy assessment unit.
- All units should audit patient choice and uptake rates for medical, surgical and conservative management of miscarriage, together with complications and failure rates.

Ectopic pregnancy

- All units should provide patient information on all aspects of ectopic pregnancy diagnosis, management and future care, together with information on future fertility.
- All early pregnancy units should record their incidence of ruptured ectopic pregnancy and of failed diagnosis of an unruptured ectopic pregnancy

Recurrent miscarriage

- All women with a history of recurrent miscarriage should be offered a follow-up visit to discuss issues such as fertility and early management of subsequent pregnancies.
- Arrangements should be in place for women with a future confirmed pregnancy test to attend an early pregnancy unit for an ultrasound scan and to receive shared antenatal care in a high-risk obstetric clinic.
- All services should audit on an annual basis adherence to the RCOG Guideline No. 17: *The Investigation and Treatment of Couples with Recurrent Miscarriage*

Infertility

- Assessment, investigation and treatment (including ovulation induction, fertility-enhancing surgery and assisted conception services) should only be carried out in secondary care centres where appropriate facilities and trained staff are available.

- The initial interview should be in private facilities and should allow for discussion with men and women together and separately as required.

Pelvic inflammatory disease

- Clear information on choice of anonymised testing, treatment and contact tracing through genitourinary medicine should be available.
- A comprehensive, integrated, community-based reproductive and sexual health walk-in service should be situated close to areas frequented by young people.
- The sexual and contraceptive service should be available in general practice, genitourinary medicine clinics and gynaecology outpatient departments.

Termination of pregnancy

- The service should have clear guidance for clinical staff to identify and respond appropriately to:
  - women at high risk of a further unplanned pregnancy
  - women undergoing termination of pregnancy without personal support
  - women under the age of 18 years
  - women with coexisting physical and psychiatric disorders and those from a disadvantaged background.
- Services should be run by teams based on national guidance which are clear about legal restrictions and be responsive to the needs of women and offer choices and preferences for method of management of abortion.
- All methods of appropriate contraception should be discussed with women at the assessment session, specifically the long-acting reversible methods of contraception for use immediately following termination of pregnancy. If this service is not available at the time of termination, then a 'fast track' system should be in place with a local family planning provider.

Female and male sterilisation

- Clear clinical and user pathways should be in place for timely referral to specialist sterilisation services. General practitioners and community specialist services should have a referral pathway with an appropriate checklist for direct access to a day-bed sterilisation unit.
- Counselling and advice on sterilisation procedures (both vasectomy and tubal occlusion) should be provided in the context of services providing a full range of information about and access to long-term reversible methods of contraception. The service must be able to demonstrate that additional care is taken in those under the age of 30 years or those without children to reduce the risk of later regret.
- There should be a lead clinician within a defined geographical area responsible for the service, governance and policy development, ensuring that governance standards are set and reported wherever procedures are undertaken and that all professionals are effectively and appropriately trained.

Diagnostic and operative hysteroscopy

- Women should have access to balanced and unbiased information leaflets before attending for diagnostic or operative hysteroscopy, including information on treatment options for menstrual problems and the services available.
- Hysteroscopic specialists must have adequate workload, review their outcome data yearly and should have attended at least one recognised meeting every 3 years.

Laparoscopic surgery

- There should be access to a suitably equipped theatre with high-quality laparoscopic video equipment for both image acquisition and recording.
- A multidisciplinary agreed protocol should be in place to treat women presenting postoperatively with possible complications related to laparoscopic surgery.
- To improve delivery of care for women with severe endometriosis, regional and national referral pathways should be developed for advanced laparoscopic procedures as the specialist centres emerge.

Heavy menstrual bleeding

- Women with heavy menstrual bleeding should have the opportunity to make informed decisions about their care and treatment, in partnership with their healthcare professionals. The treatment should aim to improve quality of life rather than focusing on menstrual blood loss alone.
- There should be a dedicated one-stop menstrual bleeding clinic with facilities within the clinic for diagnostic gynaecology, including hysteroscopy and ultrasound.
- Complications resulting from ablation, uterine artery embolisation and other treatments should be reported locally and to the National Patient Safety Agency, Medicines and Healthcare products Regulatory Agency, the uterine artery embolisation registry and other agencies as appropriate.

Menopause

- The potential long-term risks and benefits should be discussed with women before prescribing hormone replacement therapy (HRT). This discussion should be recorded in their notes, together with the indication for which HRT is prescribed.
- Locally agreed guidelines should be in place for the initial assessment and treatment of menopause in the primary care setting and referral pathways to secondary care to specialist clinics for those women who present with co-morbidity.

Urogynaecology

- There should be access to videourodynamics, ambulatory urodynamics and ultrasound facilities in the regional referral centre. Multidisciplinary team should be available at the initial consultation to minimise the patient journey to various departments.
- Combined clinics with urogynaecologists and colpoproctologists should be held to facilitate investigation and counselling of women with faecal incontinence following obstetric anal sphincter injury, and for those with bowel dysfunction in association with pelvic organ prolapse.

Benign vulval disease

- There should be dedicated vulval clinics with multidisciplinary support from dermatological, genitourinary, psychosexual and pain clinic specialists.

Colposcopy

- There should be an open explanation of expectant and surgical options. Expectant management can be offered to those women with minimal abnormalities in a cervical biopsy.
- The colposcopy clinic team should meet regularly to discuss clinic policy and guidelines. Regular meetings should also be held with cytopathologists to discuss cases of interest and difficulty.

Gynaecological oncology

- Women who have undergone radical treatment should be informed about possible long-term adverse effects and should have a clear access route to specialist help if symptoms develop.
- All patients should have a named gynaecological cancer nurse specialist and this should be clearly identified in the woman's record.
- The gynaecological cancer multidisciplinary team (MDT) requires a radiologist, clinical and medical oncologists, gynaecologists, histopathologist, specialist nurses, MDT coordinators as part of the core group. The external group should include psychologists, geneticists, palliative care specialists, and so on. Ideally, there should be more than one representative of each specialty to aid discussion. These teams must be supported with adequate administrative, secretarial, clerical and data management and information technology support.

Risk management

- Patient safety should be coordinated by a multidisciplinary risk management committee. The role of the committee should include:
  - identification, monitoring and control of risks
  - embedding continual risk assessment in all clinical areas
  - promoting awareness and understanding of patient safety issues within the unit and providing feedback.

- Users of the service should be engaged in the risk management process, for example in developing policies and protocols, systems analysis and feedback.

Gynaecological examination

- Valid patient consent should be obtained before the examination and recorded in the case notes.
- A policy should be in place to ensure a chaperone is available to assist with gynaecological examination, irrespective of the gender of the gynaecologist. The name and job title of the chaperone should be recorded in the notes.

Organisation of outpatient clinics

- It is essential that sufficient time is allowed for consultations and investigations in all settings to ensure appropriate management of the woman's clinical condition. This is especially relevant in newer settings, such as one-stop clinics, because they will be undertaking additional tasks. To ensure that future doctors are appropriately trained, the appointment system for clinics should allow adequate time for discussion between a trainee and a trainer.

Record-keeping in gynaecology

- The reports of investigations and laboratory results must be signed and dated before being filed in the notes. Any follow-up action required should be clearly annotated in the case notes.
- Processes should be in place to ensure that patients' health and other sensitive information is safeguarded against loss, damage or unauthorised access and kept confidential in accordance with the latest legislation and guidance

Index

Printed in the United States
by Baker & Taylor Publisher Services